Excavating Memory

Excavating Memory
Archaeology and Home

Elizabeth Mosier

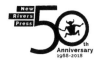

©2019 by Elizabeth Mosier
First Edition
Library of Congress Control Number: 20189602072
ISBN: 978-0-89823-382-7
e-ISBN: 978-0-89823-384-9

New Rivers Press is a nonprofit literary press associated with Minnesota State University Moorhead.

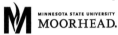

MINNESOTA STATE UNIVERSITY
MOORHEAD.

Cover and interior design by Miranda Moser
Author photo by Bill Ecklund

The publication of *Excavating Memory: Archaeology and Home* is made possible by the generous support of Minnesota State University Moorhead, the Dawson Family Endowment, and other contributors to New Rivers Press.

NRP Staff: Nayt Rundquist, Managing Editor; Kevin Carollo, Editor; Travis Dolence, Director
Thomas Anstadt, Co-Art Director; Trista Conzemius, Co-Art Director
Interns: Trevor Fellows, Laura Grimm, Kendra Johnson, Anna Landsverk, Mikaila Norman, Lauren Phillips, Ashley Thorpe, Cameron Shulz, Rachael Wing
Excavating Memory: Archaeology and Home book team: Trevor Fellows, Kendra Johnson, Cameron Schulz

 Printed in the USA on acid-free, archival-grade paper.

Excavating Memory is distributed nationally by Small Press Distribution.

New Rivers Press
c/o MSUM
1104 7th Ave S
Moorhead, MN 56563
www.newriverspress.com

For Chris

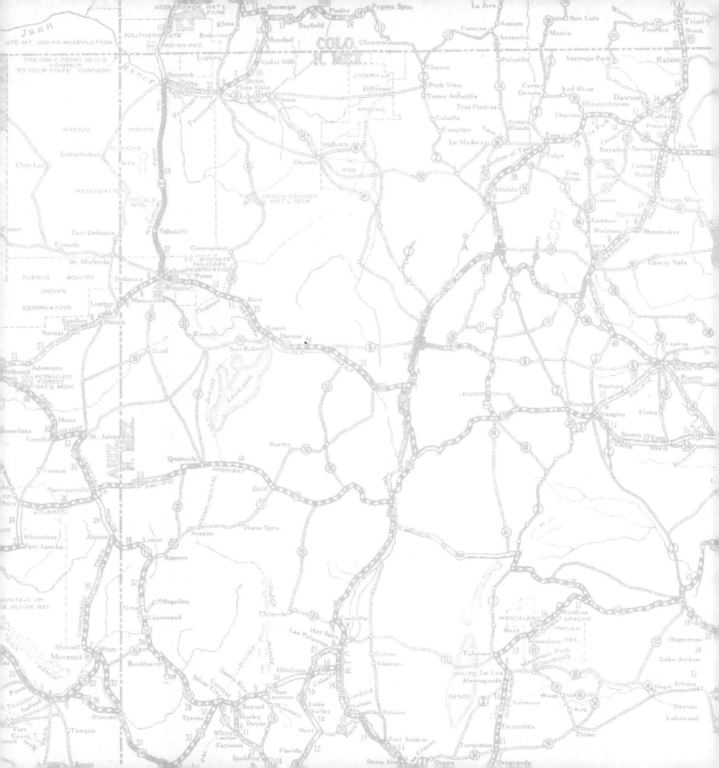

Contents

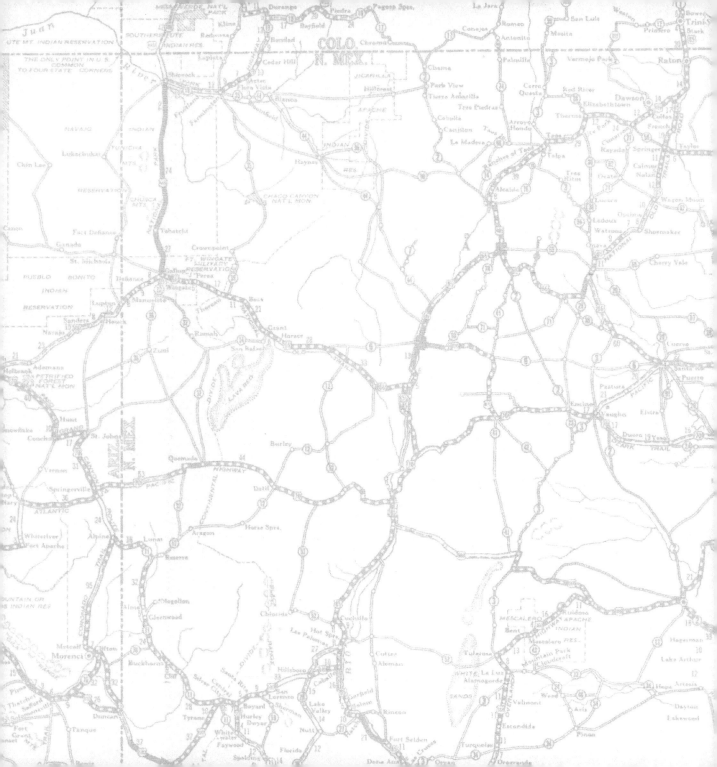

Primary Sources

1. Ephemera

I guard my cell phone number carefully, and the few people who have it know to text me, not call, since I'm usually in a classroom or driving or riding the train's Quiet Car to or from Philadelphia. *Can you pick me up? What's for dinner? Your Phillies play my Padres tonight. Got wine! Coffee at Gryphon @ 10? How was class? Math test was hard. Beautiful day! XOXO.* None of these exchanges are particularly memorable—unless made ridiculous by autocorrect—but they are important to me. These messages, spontaneous and ephemeral, are the markers of my real relationships, the moment-to-moment record of my life as it's lived.

2. Drafts

"It's a draft until you die," the poet Ellen Bryant Voigt once said. I will be reading drafts until I die: my own work, drafts written by the elementary school kids I teach through the Pennsylvania Young Writers Day program, the teenagers I mentor, my Bryn Mawr College students, my writer friends, and the adults enrolled in my evening workshops. I love the promise and playfulness of a draft, which little kids intuitively understand. When I'm with third graders, we fracture fairy tales, beginning not with "Once upon a time" but instead with "In the days before iPhones." Not "in a land far, far away" but "in the corner of the closet where the lost things live." Not "there lived a princess" but "there lived a troll named Terrible, who tried to be kind." The kids put these odd pieces together in outra-

Elizabeth Mosier

geous, often hilarious, original forms. Fairy tales teach us how time and telling changes a story—how, when we break with tradition, we incorporate traces of the past and present, even as we progress to something new. What lasts? What's left behind?

3. Diaries

My mother was diagnosed with Alzheimer's disease in 2007. Her datebooks from 2003–08, recovered when I spent a week in my childhood home sorting through the flotsam of our family history, tell a heartbreaking story of her mental decline. Within their pages is proof that—despite my mother's angry, fearful protests that her mind was still intact—she used strategies to preserve what she couldn't remember: check marks for medications she'd already taken, black *X*s drawn through the days as they passed. A year after she made her last entry, my mother would not recognize me—could not make sense of my face, my voice, my hand placed on her arm. But here, on my birthday in 2008, there is a note in her graceful handwriting: Call Lib. And from that ink mark on the page arises a picture: the pen in her fingers, her hand brushing the paper, my smart and beautiful and unlucky mother making her plans, accounting for her days.

4. Documents

"My dear Johny, It is with great grief I have to acquaint thee, that thy precious brother is taken with the disorder . . ."

So begins the letter dated September 20, 1798, from Philadelphian Caleb Cresson Sr. to his son John Elliott, delivered by a servant named Glasgow to a home in Upper Dublin Township, Montgomery County, just outside the contagious city. The "disorder" he doesn't name is Yellow Fever, which Caleb Sr. and Caleb Jr. would survive, but which many residents of Cresson's Square (the dense block of tenements this prominent Quaker developed for mid-century immigrants behind his three-story "plainly finished" house at 43 Cherry Street) would not.

This letter, part of Haverford College's collection, brings me into the sick room where "my dear Caleb had not the usual pains in the head and back as violent as some, the pukeing was considerable." It places me close to Mother—who is opening the windows to let in fresh air, wiping the floor with vinegar, urging Caleb Jr. to drink tamarind and lemon water —even as two centuries of medical knowledge distance me from the scene, even as I wince at the treatment described as "by Mercury altogether, without bleeding or sweating."

2

This letter has been preserved because it was written by a city leader and captures a significant event in history. But I read it to find the shadows behind the surface drama, the evidence of other men and women who lived and loved and died on the same ground that is, today, the vast lawn of the National Constitution Center. I read it for the 1865 footnote added by Caleb Sr.'s descendant, Charles C. Cresson: "... Glasgow was a big fat coloured man—a servant . . . who married a white woman, but it was kept secret till after Glasgow's death when she came and kissed him as he laid in his coffin."

5. *Artifacts*

As a volunteer technician at Philadelphia's Independence National Historical Park Archeology Laboratory, I help to wash, label, mend, and catalogue the more than one million artifacts recovered from the National Constitution Center site that includes Cresson's Square. Processing these fragments of colonial history, I am learning to "read" artifacts —that is, to look for the potter's thumbprint in the rolled rim of the redware vessel, to tell a pig's tooth from a cow's, to understand how an object accrues and loses meaning and value in different physical and temporal contexts.

The Cresson's Alley tenants—laborers, tobacconists, bakers, printers—shared one large multi-seat privy pit for five tenement buildings, so it's impossible to pair an artifact to a particular person one-to-one. Still, the objects discarded there long ago communicate to us today. They tell us, for instance, that kids' cups and coin banks taught the concept of private property, while temperance-themed transferware pitchers embedded the message of sober industry. Then, as now, what and how much was eaten, as well as how the dish was prepared, delineated social classes. Recovered animal remains reveal that the merchant class preferred birds, while the laboring class ate fish. Everyone ate pigs, it seems. In Feature 193, the privy pit once used by eighteenth-century German baker Godfrey Minnick, a pig's tooth was found among sherds of glazed pearlware china and a glass tumbler embossed with the word *Liberty*.

All this digging and processing of primary sources creates a record of life that is both detailed and fragmented, much like memory.

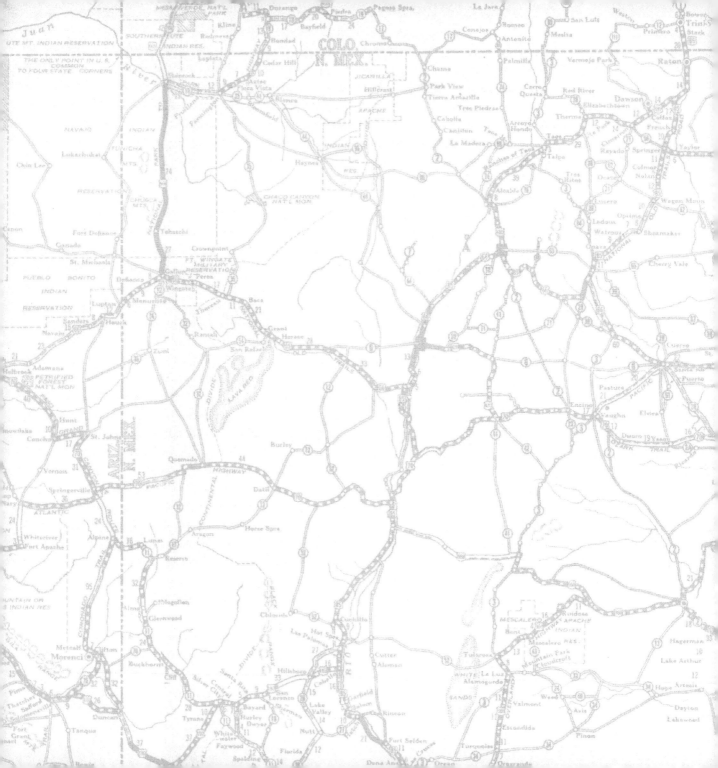

Cinéma Vérité

April 16, 1972. The United States launched Apollo 16 and bombed the Haiphong port in Vietnam. President Nixon met with Henry Kissinger and Major John Brennan before calling the Reverend Billy Graham for counsel. Gloria Steinem prepared to launch the first issue of *Ms.* I attended my friend Shelly's ninth birthday party, an event that is the pin in the map of my late-boomer childhood in Phoenix, Arizona—a long trip from JFK to Reagan, from Love-In to trickle-down, from the elevation of mothers (then called "home economists") to their trivialization as "stay-at-home moms."

That day, I parked my banana-seat bike against the Smiths' stockade fence and entered the backyard carnival. There, I tossed coins at Dixie cups floating in a water-filled wheelbarrow, shot baskets granny style, wildly over-guessed my weight (as confirmed by a bathroom scale), "soaked the clown" (Shelly's good sport little sister peeking through a curtain) with a wet sponge, and played Twister tentatively in the prissy dress my mom made me wear, while the other girls moved easily in culottes and hot pants.

Mr. Smith, wearing first-wave hipster glasses, tallied our points for each carnival game. After lunch and cake, we lined up in ranked order to choose a prize from a row of stuffed animals made out of bright-colored fabric, which dangled from strings across the patio. I noticed that the rhinoceros matched the cute blue-and-yellow striped jumpsuit Shelly had worn on picture day—a clue that Mrs. Smith, the party's mastermind, had sewn the stuffed animals herself.

I was awed. To me, Shelly's homemade party was magical. I took it all in and kept it close, a talisman to ward off my vague shame about being a latchkey kid: my playground nickname "Women's Lib"; friends whispering, "Their house is always messy," when they came over to play; Mom's new suits and clack-clack heels on the sidewalk and the spring in her step when she left our apartment to sell houses. Even my young, single fourth-grade teacher would ridicule the revolution the following year, buzzing the term "Ms." so it stung. But already, I could see that my dad was off the hook, while my working mother was vulnerable to criticism.

Though Mom was my role model, I secretly wanted to be Mrs. Smith. I pictured myself as a grownup not selling houses but making things, the way Mrs. Smith made cool clothes and crafts and that wonderful backyard carnival.

Over the years, I recalled Shelly's birthday party so many times I risked forgetting it, as the memory became symbolic for something I couldn't quite name, and the symbol threatened to obliterate my experience. And then, decades later, I found myself in my own backyard, pinning calico prairie bonnets to a clothesline—the prizes I'd managed to make, despite my directional dyslexia, for my young daughter's pioneer-themed birthday party. Seeing the colorful bonnets twist gently in the breeze made me suddenly stop where I was, startled by the force of my old childhood longing.

As a child, envy of other families made me shy, so I didn't share my appreciation for Shelly's party with her until just before our thirty-year high school reunion, when I emailed her a picture of the prairie bonnets I'd made and cited her mom as the source of my creative inspiration. Shelly wrote back immediately. She'd found the old home movie of that birthday party and converted it to a .mov file, she said. It was attached if I wanted to take a look.

I didn't remember being filmed. Unlike my daughters' highly documented childhoods, mine is archived mostly in memory, fact-checked against diary entries and letters, annual class and team photos, and scattered shots of Christmas mornings and family vacations at the beach or Disneyland. It wasn't until a year after Shelly's party that Craig Gilbert's ground-breaking documentary, *An American Family*, aired, alerting us to the concept of life as performance, to the camera's role as catalyst for drama, and to the issue of how editing cuts away complexity to craft caricature.

But even then, we couldn't have anticipated an era in which our lives looped back to us incessantly through social media and reality TV—the landscape in which the video of Shelly's birthday party arrived in my email inbox, an unearthed time capsule.

I sat staring at my laptop screen for a long time, afraid to open the file and play the old reel. I was remembering the time my mother and I visited a strip mall antique store on her day off—how excited she'd been to hunt for old treasures, and how disappointed she'd looked as we walked the air-conditioned aisles, surveying the salvaged past. Not long after that, Alzheimer's disease cleared the place in my mother's brain where her daughter had once lived. I worried that time might have tumbled my own memories smooth, distorting experience by making it ideal. But mostly, at midlife, I feared the record of reality might rob me of this small remembered joy.

Finally, though, I couldn't resist.

"Shelly's 9th Birthday" is eight minutes, sixteen seconds, of unedited film footage capturing details so familiar that my memory hadn't flagged them (a garden hose filling the evaporating swimming pool, whitewash sunscreen painted on the trunks of citrus trees), events that had gained meaning with time (the sudden cut to an airplane flying overhead, still a novelty in 1972), and images I reviewed with new empathy. There, again, was that nine-year-old girl overdressed for the party, watching the others and nervously chewing her nails. I knew her instantly. All these years later, I knew her mother, too: my mother, like me, at work before her children woke, counting on appearances to keep others' judgment at bay.

Mrs. Smith's homemade stuffed animals were just as I'd remembered them—not corrupted into metaphor, the writers' consolation prize. As if I'd shot the film myself, the camera lingered over each one in turn: cat, snake, hen, rhino, bunny, bear, and frog with the yellow belly and button eyes. That last one—the smallest prize—was mine. I can't recall where I stood in the carnival game tally, but I remember choosing it because my mom liked frogs.

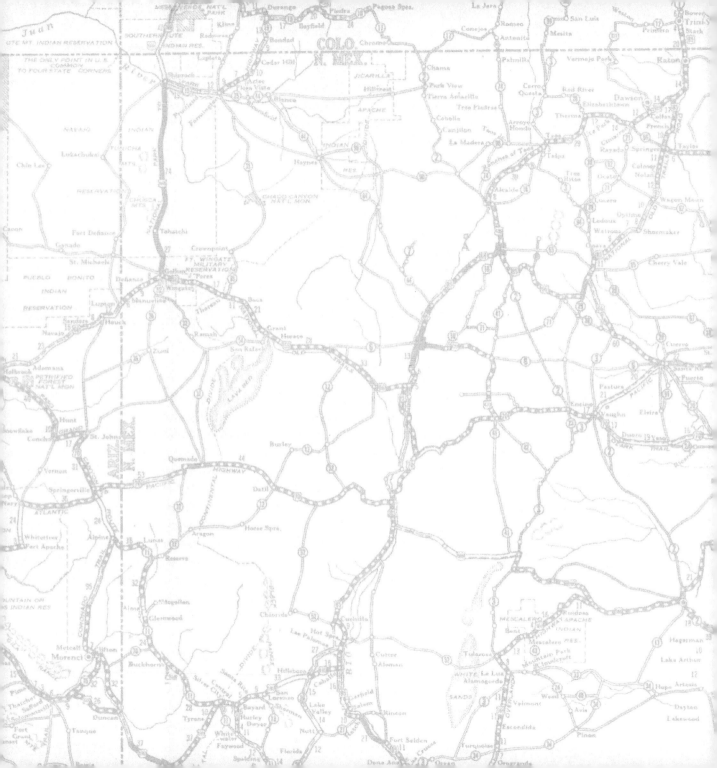

Art and Artifact

"Writers are archaeologists," I tell the fourth-grade class at New Garden Elementary School in Toughkenamon, Pennsylvania, where I'm visiting for their annual Young Writers Day. "We dig up a piece of our experience and study it, and then we put what we've learned into words."

This metaphor I use with the kids actually comes from my life: many years of washing, labeling, repairing, and cataloguing the contents of Old City Philadelphia's colonial privy pits as a volunteer at the Independence National Historical Park Archeology Lab. There, I learned that the point of urban archaeology isn't to preserve the artifacts recovered from the ground, as I'd always thought, but rather to learn about people from what they threw away. I learned that archaeology is every bit as tedious and absorbing as writing, involving a process that is as valuable as its product. Because I teach writing from my own practice, I bring this hands-on lesson to the classroom today.

I show the students "artifacts" found in my junk drawers and in my husband's art studio: an antique key fob from the Warwick Hotel in Rittenhouse Square, a cart wheel, a paint sponge, a brass button embossed with an eagle, a palm-sized sock monkey, and a blob of melted aluminum shaped like a T-Rex or a praying woman, depending on which way it's turned. The kids are bouncing in their seats, raising their hands, reaching for the objects like they're prizes. This, in a snapshot, is the difference between teaching in college and in elementary school: I don't have to remind these kids how to play.

Through this game I don't call writing, students practice literary skills: observing something closely, like scientists, and using sensory detail and simile to describe what they've found. To play is to experiment. Just as we aim to get better by practicing a sport or an instrument, putting experience into words lets us test what we know and then try again, in order to come closer to writing the truth.

At the lab where I volunteer, I'm inspired by the archaeologists' dedication to their practice, evident in the care with which they account for every last button and seed bead, slowly fashioning stories from their findings. The writer's job is similar. It takes time to dig deep, to reexamine old artifacts of meaning we once accepted as valid so that we can, eventually, get the story right—or, to put it another way, get the story less wrong.

* * *

I love visiting New Garden, which is a quarter tank of gas and a world away from my suburban Philadelphia neighborhood. On my way here, I passed old stone houses and faded red barns that confirm Chester County's horsey-set stereotype, and farmed fields and bright-painted *taquerías* that counter it. Inside the school, the halls are filled with tempera self-portraits of pink and brown faces and the pungent scent of fertilizer from the mushroom farms nearby. In the Kennett Consolidated School District, one in five employed people works in agriculture, including Mexican immigrants with American-born children who attend district schools. The school's newsletter is two-sided, its *Noticias de la Directora* printed in both English and Spanish.

I'm happy to be here, at home in this classroom of children named Marisol and Miguel and Javier—maybe because my hometown of Phoenix, Arizona, feels more and more distant these days. I'm lucky to be traveling with this band of writers brought together by Mary Beth Lauer, the founder of Pennsylvania Young Writers Day. Teaching writing teaches me. Every time I step into a classroom, I'm reminded that a writer's practice is about more than publishing.

In teams, the kids study their chosen artifacts by tracing them, sniffing them, tapping them on the desktop, turning them over, and tossing them up in the air. I circle the room, studying the kids—taking note of ponytails, buzz cuts, and Bieber-sweeps; pink-painted fingernails and nails bitten to the quick; t-shirts honoring Phillies players and popular brands; two-dozen variations on the unofficial school uniform of sneakers and jeans. But these details tell me more about the pressures of the school context than they do about any particular kid. I can't know them just by looking. I need to hear their words.

"Now pretend it's fifty years from now," I say, "and you've found these things on the playground. Who left them here? What are they? Were they lost or thrown away or buried here for a reason? How? Why?"

Then we're off and running. From these questions arise character, setting, and conflict: the seedlings of the tales these kids will tell. Proof that in a plugged-in world, imagination still thrives; proof, too, that collaboration changes a story. As the student groups plant and prune various plot lines, one member—not necessarily the most talkative or the one with the neatest penmanship, but rather, the one known as the best listener—scribbles away, recording.

I've shown the same set of objects to hundreds of students at dozens of schools over the years, and I haven't heard the same story twice. This variety no longer surprises me, though it always amazes me. As these young writers observe and reflect and give voice to their discoveries, like all of us, they bring their unique ways of seeing, their interests, and their biases to their storytelling. Listening to them read their different versions aloud, I picture a line of kids extending from the past into the future, passing these objects from hand to hand, assessing what's important, what's useful, what's worth keeping. And I'm struck again by how the words we choose to tell a story—our own, our family's, our community's, our country's—make history, an account that, some day, generations after ours will tell about who we are now.

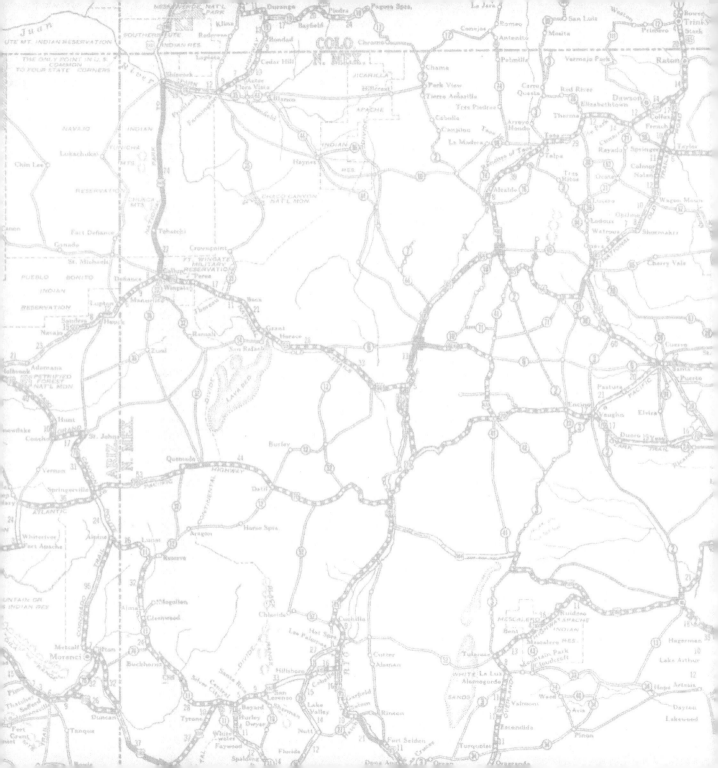

The Phoenix Indian School

My high school was next door to the Phoenix Indian School. As a freshman, I played softball with my team on our south field, which was separated from their boarding school by a flimsy hurricane fence. Sometimes, we'd see a few Native American boys there, their fingers hooked through the wire as they silently watched us play, but we never spoke to each other.

This border fence—and the nearby street named Indian School Road—marked the limit of what I knew about the school. Not until 1991, when the Indian School's closing coincided with my writerly interest in my hometown, did I research the educational system designed to make many tribes into one and, through enforced assimilation to Anglo culture, to make Native Americans disappear. The so-called "assimilation era" ended in the 1930s, and the Indian School curriculum was reformed to teach academic subjects and not just basic trades. But the words of U.S. Commissioner of Indian Affairs Thomas Morgan, in 1891, are irrevocably and shamefully part of the school's foundation: "It's cheaper to educate Indians than to kill them."

Artifacts help tell the story. Before Steele Indian School Park was opened on the site in 2001, city archaeologists excavated the contents of a 230' x 165' trash dump very near where my team had fouled a few balls. Among the tools of assimilation abandoned there between 1891–1926 were the porcelain heads of white dolls used to socialize girls and rusted steam whistles that blasted at intervals to teach students the concept of clock time.

Elizabeth Mosier

But there was also evidence of resistance: forbidden fetishes and pottery sherds smuggled from home; flaked stone points showing off students' carving skills and the broken dining hall plates on which they practiced; a cache of unlabeled combs, violating school policy that taught hygiene and the concept of personal property. These artifacts are beautifully subversive—ironic imagery in a landscape where the captives were compelled to trade tribal clothing for uniforms, native languages for English, the Native American we for the American I.

* * *

So many stories beneath the ground, I thought as I walked through the re-imagined Steele Indian School Park on a November night the year my father died. Back in Phoenix for Hospice of the Valley's community memorial service in the park, I took a last look around before I joined my family on the grass. We sat together in the dark, surrounded by hundreds of other grieving people, all of us quietly waiting and watching, as images of our loved ones flashed on a giant screen and then were gone.

The Big Tree, Phoenix, Arizona

The Big Tree was already old when we were kids at Madison Meadows Elementary School in Phoenix, Arizona, and it was wide enough to block the path from home to away-from-home. The leaves of the towering eucalyptus laced the sky; sunburnt bark peeled and fell away from its body; its roots gripped the ground where it had stood for at least a half-century. The tree, a native Australian transplanted by Arizona pioneers, gave shade and cover for the fights that began in our schoolyard and smoldered in class until the last bell. We all understood what "Meet me at the Big Tree" meant. The words were a challenge, a red flag signaling to the crowd of bike-straddling students to gather and witness and fan the flames.

Beneath the Big Tree, we watched boys—sometimes best friends—wrestle murderously in the dirt. We saw a girl's tube top slip to her ribs as, bare-breasted, she pummeled the boy who'd broken her heart. Some of us kissed or smoked or drank beer there, and some of us just said we did. I chickened out of kissing the boy I secretly loved—a Huck Finn character of confusing parentage who courted me with gifts (a dented wooden ruler; a citrus-scented eraser; a palm-sized, half-deflated Phoenix Suns basketball) before dropping the invitation on my desk one day on his way to the water fountain: FIRST BASE AFTER SCHOOL. I didn't have to ask him where. The venue was understood.

Just down the road from our K–8 school, the Big Tree was the center of our circle, both a battleground and a retreat. As we got older and tested our boundaries, it was our midnight meeting place, a familiar springboard to new experiences. This was way before cell phones, so we couldn't text or call each other with our whereabouts. Hearts pounding, we'd hide behind the tree's massive trunk until we heard our co-conspirators whistle the code. Then we'd emerge and roam our neighborhood together in the dark, studying the skeletons of our houses illuminated from the inside, and our backyard swimming pools gone still and quiet, reflecting the moon.

Once, I met my father at the Big Tree to strategize in secret after my mother—angry and scared as her diseased brain dissolved to lace—became violent, bruising Dad's back and breaking his thumb. But that happened many years later, long after I'd grown up and left behind my childhood in Phoenix, or thought I had.

The houses in our North Central neighborhood, called Orangewood, were a storybook collection of pretty revivals (American and Spanish Colonial, Pueblo, Tudor, and English Cottage) mixed in with more typical California Ranchers, long and low and land-grabbing. These domiciles were just stage dressing, though. In the Valley of the Sun, we didn't know the insides of our friends' houses as well as we did the outdoor spaces we all shared: the mountain parks, bike trails, and Murphy's bridle path lined with graceful olive and ash trees; the Madison Meadows School bleachers, basketball courts, and playing fields; the citrus orchards, the stand of giant eucalyptus trees along the Arizona Canal, and the lone Big Tree.

The mountains around us (North and South, the White Tanks, Camelback, and Squaw Peak, now officially called Piestewa) were our compass points, orienting us in space and to geography. This was helpful, even comforting. In our air-conditioned neighborhood of green lawns, sparkling pools, non-native trees, and imported architecture, it was all too easy to forget where we were. Sometimes we had to look to the mountains—find the nimble silhouette of a saguaro cactus thriving in the Mars-like landscape—or smell the rainy-day scent of a creosote bush to remember that we lived in the Sonoran Desert. When I return to Phoenix now, I still search for these natural features to find my way amid all the traffic and commerce and new, bland, gated communities.

The disorientation we felt was by design. In Phoenix, desert denial is a survival strategy, a sales tactic, even a point of civic pride. Though the view outside our art class window was of blinding sunshine and skinny date palms, we were instructed to sketch stylish snowmen and bright autumn leaves falling from deciduous trees. In winter, when the dead grass sparkled with morning frost, we squinted and saw white fields of snow; we scraped up the scant crystals to fling at each other, mimicking snowball fights we'd seen in children's books and our parents' photo albums. Before water parks were popular, Phoenix had the first faux beach. Big Surf, its engine designed by my father's company, used basic toilet technology to flush 2.5 million gallons of water into waves at three-minute intervals.

By defying the desert in these absurd ways, we were following a long tradition that began in 1867. That's when an ex-Confederate cavalryman, Jack Swilling, looked out across the arid valley abandoned by the Hohokam Indians and imagined a modern Phoenix rising from verdant land irrigated by the tribe's clever system of canals.

It turns out that the promise of a second chance is powerful motivation to move. And what better setting for rebirth than a city resurrected from the ashes of an ancient civilization, a mecca enabled (if not sustained) by Swilling's new and improved plan to channel the Salt River's flow? Our city's population tripled in the time it took us to graduate from high school, and it has doubled again since then. Eventually, one and a half million people would journey to Phoenix seeking cheap land or dry air, employment or an education, to get lost in the sprawling metropolis or to find themselves there.

But these pilgrims, including our parents, didn't leave their old lives behind. They didn't prepare physically or mentally for hardship, or give themselves up to this strange new site where their personal transformation would take place. Rather, they came to Phoenix and built an ice factory. They diverted the Salt and Gila Rivers, paved the desert, and planted rose bushes They created a theme park called Legend City, which replicated the landscape in miniature and presented our history to us as myth. Some of us had never been to the Grand Canyon, but we'd been to Legend City to ride kid-scale ore cars through the haunted "Lost Dutchman's Mine" (believed to be hidden within Arizona's Superstition Mountains) and take a boat trip down the "River of Legends," filthy with animal waste runoff from the nearby Phoenix Zoo. In social studies class at school, we never seemed to get past the Civil War, but the River of Legends took us to "Cchise's Stronghold" in the Chiricahua Mountains, where stiff-armed Apaches staged a shootout with a troop of cavalrymen that looked like they'd been fashioned from castoff department store mannequins.

By the time we were old enough to learn the dictionary definition of "irony," Phoenix had grown into an unsustainable city of golf courses and resort hotels featuring continuously running man-made fountains that flowed into lovely sculpted basins and evaporated into the air. No wonder we were called to the Big Tree. Giant and incongruous, it was to us a vestige of the natural landscape, a survivor that had withstood heat and limb-breaking winds, and that had witnessed our adolescent wars.

The irony is that the eucalyptus isn't natural in Phoenix; the Australian import competes with, and can destroy, Arizona's native species, and it's highly flammable besides. That's a problem in a hot, dry city with a single-digit dew point temperature for most of the year, where the summer monsoon season brings wind and rain and lightning.

Still, the Big Tree, with its deep roots and tall branches, is a potent symbol for all of us, even after all these years. It stands, weathered and defiant, a conduit between earth and sky, body and spirit.

* * *

A few years ago, on a tour of the battlefield at Gettysburg with my childhood friend Laurie, who was visiting from Chicago, our guide wisely skipped the monuments and battle plans and tailored his talk to our teenage daughters. "Right there," he said, pointing to the house-turned-field-hospital, "the limbs discarded after surgery were piled right up to the sill of the first-floor windows. Imagine the gauntlet those brave volunteer nurses, most of them completely inexperienced, had to walk through just to go to work." He told us about a young woman who enlisted (and cross-dressed) as a Union soldier, and about another, Tillie Pierce, who wrote about the battle in her published diary. He implored us to imagine the sticky summer heat, the air dark with cannon smoke, the line of Philadelphians holding ground on Cemetery Ridge as the Confederates made their slow-mo march—Pickett's charge—across a field of last resort.

As he recounted the men's hellish, doomed journey, goosebumps rose along my arm. I wasn't just reacting to being at the legendary battlefield, hearing the zealot guide's stories filled with gruesome details—but also to the summer heat, the light breeze on my bare arms, the reunion with my old friend, and the sudden awareness that each of us was now mother to two girls like the girls we'd been way back when. I was feeling what G. M. Trevelyan called "the poetry of history," which, as he says, "lies in the quasi-miraculous fact that once, on this earth, once, on this familiar spot of ground, walked other men and women, as actual as we are today, thinking their own thoughts, swayed by their own passions, but now all gone, one generation vanishing into another, gone as utterly as we ourselves shall shortly be gone." That day, our guide's stories brought history close and held us to the spot listening, while lightning flashed in a distant corner of the darkening sky, heralding an afternoon storm that would fell the last Civil War witness tree in the National Cemetery.

My daughter took a picture of it. I thought of the Big Tree.

Certain artifacts from our pasts are discarded; others stay with us, charged with emotional power. I visit the Big Tree every time I'm in Phoenix; from my desk, I search for the God's-eye view of it on Google Maps. The tree often appears in my stories and essays, as itself or in disguise. I've imagined my fictional characters standing beneath the protective umbrella of its branches (where, in my memory, the air tastes of coconut and citrus, sweat and cooling mud), their hearts beating loudly from danger they've summoned, as they swagger and posture, daring an enemy or defender or life itself to strike the first blow.

But the stories we tell ourselves affect us, too; they become part of our personal mythology. The boy whose kiss I once refused was gone before we turned twenty-one. And the friends (boys then, now men) who witnessed his death by self-inflicted gunshot wound are still making their way back home from that awful night. When I met my father at the Big Tree—the location chosen unconsciously, unintentionally—I pleaded with him to see what my brothers and I saw, that taking care of our poor mother was killing him.

That night, I pocketed a large piece of the Big Tree's bark—one that curved gracefully, like a hand at rest or half a prayer—and carried it home with me to Philadelphia. This tree bark now sits on my desk as I sort through the story of my mother's decline and my father's rescue. Occasionally, I stop writing and rest my hand on the wood and, in the mysterious way that memory frees and fails us, I'm a teenager again. I am returned like magic to some lost sense of safety, as I kneel beneath the Big Tree and touch its rough trunk, and feel its old, gnarled roots beneath my sneakers.

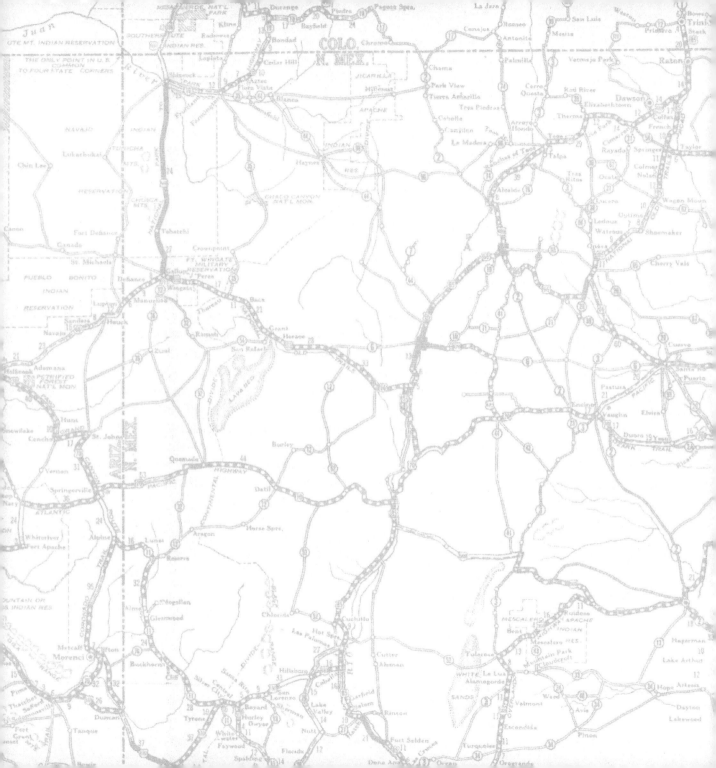

My Mother's Books

The summer before I left home for Bryn Mawr College, my mother gave me two things: my first serious wool coat, mail-ordered from Talbot's back east, and a list of books I should have read by that point in my life.

The coat was classic and elegant and perfectly ugly, I thought—my mother's idea of a Bryn Mawr woman striding purposefully to the library to translate a passage from ancient Greek. Of course I had to hate it; I was seventeen, and still had trouble untangling my mother's taste and ambition from my own. Even my decision about college was corrupted by her favor. Bryn Mawr was my first choice, but first, it was my mother's choice for me.

The list is three pages long, single-spaced, recorded in my mother's neat, slanted script. There's something old-fashioned about her handwriting, which reveals the untroubled faith that allowed her to create a literary canon for me by consulting no higher authority than the floor-to-ceiling bookshelves in our living room. She listed the authors and their works alphabetically, leaving no room between their names for additions or debate.

I knew that my mother's list, like my fancy education, was intended to help me surpass her. I understood, too, that I would never catch up. I am an avid but turtle-slow reader, unable to take in words on a page without listening for their music or wondering about the author's choices or revising sentences in my head. My mother, by comparison, doesn't read books—she devours them. In my memory, she wears an apron over her business suit as she stands in front of the bookshelves making her list, as if to protect her clothing from her voracious appetite for words.

I find now that I've filed the list under "Résumé," that dropsafe of things I've done to enable a writing career or perhaps, at times, to avoid one. My mother, who couldn't help imploring me occasionally to take a job with tangible benefits, used to give me a new business suit every Christmas—either to flatter herself or to save me from downward mobility. But she also gave me what amounts to her résumé in the form of a personal syllabus. As if the true measure of success is not what one has done, but rather, what one has read.

This image of my mother at her bookshelves is almost like a religious symbol to me. I conjure it when I need to ward off a bleaker vision of unread books piling up in warehouses, their jackets torn and bodies remaindered. Whatever my mother intended when she gave me her list, she conveyed to me the certainty that the life of a writer is a worthwhile pursuit. In that way, she sent me off to school wrapped up in something dignified and durable, better able than that tasteful wool coat from Talbot's to keep out the cold.

I Have,
I Fear, he
Literary Temperament

February 28, 1920, gray, cold, dull
"I used to feel that having big thoughts and feeling deeply were a sign of greatness and that I was marked, so to speak. Query: Can I write? Is this an indication of the good taste of Bryn Mawr or my vile style?"

These words, written by Bryn Mawr College freshman Dorothy Burr Thompson, Class of 1923, remind me of my own adolescent musings, source material for my first published novel. When I wrote the book, I'd just begun teaching creative writing at Bryn Mawr in the same building where I'd once met with my Freshman English professor to discuss the many flaws in my weekly critical papers. Fifteen years later, the psychological landscape of the campus was different because I was different; in order to access the awe and insecurity I'd felt as a student, I had to excavate my past.

I dug up my old fears and failures (detailed in the journals I kept from 1980–84) as well as my grand plans and successes (headlined in letters home) in order to remember what I thought and felt at seventeen. Only in retrospect can I plot my career as a coherent series of events along a rising action line leading to an MFA in creative writing and work as a writer and teacher. As if this were the inevitable conclusion to a story of a girl from Phoenix who studied psychology and planned to earn a PhD in the field.

Dorothy Burr Thompson did the opposite; she entered Bryn Mawr as a writer (she'd penned poems and stories and a novel draft, *Marjorie*, at Miss Hill's School in

Philadelphia) and exited as a renowned scholar of classical archaeology. As I learned from her *New York Times* obituary, she graduated *summa cum laude*, specialized in ancient terra cotta art, and lived to be 101. Knowing what Dorothy had accomplished in her long, productive, fruitful career diffuses some of the narrative tension in her life story. But for me, this answer to the question of how she made use of her education only brought the query she'd penned in her 1919–23 diaries—*Can I write?*—into greater relief. I remember asking myself the same question in college. My students, in conference, often ask it of me.

Dorothy could write. In fact, she published more than fifty scholarly papers and books on her excavation work in Athens. Her life-spanning diaries in the Bryn Mawr College Archives reveal that she wrote fiction and poetry into her forties, and yet this work isn't even mentioned in her obituary. This omission troubled me. Perhaps seeing how a complex life with conflicting ambitions might be abstracted to fit an archive box or a column of type is what directed my attention to the subtext of Dorothy's story: her literary aspirations and the role our shared alma mater played in altering the arc of her life.

* * *

Monday, September 22, 1919
"Four years of college should prove whether I have a right to write or should take up a manlier way of life."

Bryn Mawr College, founded in 1885 by pragmatic Quakers (and shaped by its formidable first dean and second president, M. Carey Thomas, who set the agenda for "solid and scientific" instruction), was in some ways an unlikely choice for a young woman who declared herself a "literary type." With its rigorous curriculum and graduate schools, Bryn Mawr broadcast its academic mission as the first American institution where women could earn the PhD degree. Creative writing was not yet part of the curriculum. And practically speaking, the long list of required courses in—English, philosophy, math, science, Greek, Latin, and two modern languages—left Dorothy even less time for outlining her new novel (working title: *Youth*) than I would have six decades later, as I fulfilled slightly less onerous divisional and foreign language requirements.

Like Dorothy, I felt the pressure of Bryn Mawr's mission, but thanks to the women who came before me, I never felt I had to "take up a manlier way of life" to justify my education there. I chose a women's college, in part, so that I could forget that I was female. For four years, I was free of the qualifier that so often came with any accolade: "That's good (work or reasoning or writing) for a girl."

When Dorothy matriculated in 1919 (post-armistice, pre-suffrage), Bryn Mawr still had much to prove about what women and women's colleges could do. Reading between the lines of Dorothy's diary entries, it seemed to me that Bryn Mawr—M. Carey Thomas embodied in Collegiate Gothic architecture—was the perfect dramatic setting for the personal conflict Dorothy identified in her diary: would she be an artist or an academic? Though her fateful meeting with then-President Thomas wouldn't occur until Dorothy was a sophomore, Thomas was already an antagonist of sorts in the internal struggle that intensified during Dorothy's undergraduate years.

* * *

August 8, 1920 clear, warm, soft
"Oh, such a soft summer day, peaceful and dreary, ill fit for recording turbulent and petty feelings! Yet I must. I have, I fear, the literary temperament—capable of being happy only in writing, however foolish may be my ideas. Every day I have promised myself an orgy in the empty inviting blank book . . ."

By sophomore year, though Dorothy laments being "gradually weighed down by study to less artistic tasks," she begins using her diary as a writer does: to practice her craft and articulate her emerging literary aesthetic. Her entries change in content and style; self-analysis becomes literary criticism (she admires Jane Austen and Ivan Turgenev) and ruminations on her friendships turn to development of her characters. "Malcolm is dead," she writes on September 13, 1920—and I have to re-read the passage several times before I understand that Malcolm is not a friend or family member, but her fictional creation. "Perhaps it is wrong," she adds, "or rather, inadvisable, to suffer so much for an imaginary pain . . ." Her entries from this year reflect new awareness of herself as a protagonist in a story of collegiate self-invention. In one passage, she refers to her eponymous first novel when she reflects, "I always knew Marjorie was myself."

Again and again in her diaries, Dorothy pits the "literary type" (such as her brilliant friend D.W., to whom she "confided all my schemes and hopes") against the "scientific personality" (typified by her math professor, Anna Pell). She pursues these women's divergent stories as a novelist does, perhaps seeking resolution to her personal conflict. By spring of sophomore year, D.W. makes the "upper ten" for the European Fellowship that Dorothy covets; by spring of junior year, she withdraws from Bryn Mawr after suffering a "nervous breakdown." Dorothy's wariness is informed by these dramatic events, which reinforce her own associations: inspiration with depression, dullness with mental and physical health. Throughout her diaries, she expresses this dichotomous view, but never as succinctly as in her entry on February 28, 1920: "I'd write tonight, but curiously, I feel vigorous, but uninspired, like a strong cow."

On December 21, 1920, Dorothy presents (in dialogue with stage directions) a pointed conversation with "Miss P" that takes place in her home, called "Yarrow." As the two women speak, Anna Pell's odd, "dog-like" husband Alexander shuffles in and out of the room, muttering that his wife is "crazy" and that he and she are "incompatible equations."

> *D—Why am I more stupid as I go on?*
> *Miss P—Misdirected energy, Miss Burr.*
> *D—Must one give up everything, and health?*
> *Miss P—Almost (pathetically but unsentimentally). You must make a great many sacrifices; it is an isolated life. You can't talk about your work to any one. But Mathematicians don't consider—they go straight ahead. (Bursting through reserve.) It's the most wonderful thing in the world.*

A month later, on January 27, 1921, Dorothy depicts another visit to Anna Pell at Yarrow to deliver a puzzle she's promised to bring. "Her eyes were red and swollen and her face white," she notes, signaling an important scene with slower pacing and sensory detail. "I was embarrassed to meet her, so I chatted jauntily on about Miss Blake, engines, puzzles, etc. trying to set on myself as theatrical and romantic in imagining that she had been crying." Mrs. Pell takes the puzzle, though her manner is odd, and Dorothy feels unwelcome. "I got out quickly," she reflects, as she builds to her point, "without knowing exactly why."

Later, she's shocked to learn from another professor that Alexander Pell had died from a stroke just that morning. "That that provincial, untrivial, earnest woman should have received me so undramatically, even tho' she was in undoubted sorrow . . . a few hours after her husband's death—is a triumph of the scientific personality," she concludes. "A literary woman could not have been so matter of fact."

Dorothy presents the scene as more evidence of her own different temperament, but her writing also reveals an instinct for characterization. As it turns out, her portrait of the strange Mr. Pell was prescient. More than eighty years later, author Richard Pipes would make the case in *The Degaev Affair: Terror and Treason in Tsarist Russia* that "Alexander Pell" was in fact notorious Russian terrorist Sergei Degaev, accomplice to the murder of Tsar Alexander II, leading a secret double life as the husband of Bryn Mawr's math department chair.

Now that's a story—one Dorothy might have written.

Sophomore year was a turning point for Dorothy, as it was for me. That year, my Developmental Psychology professor noted that my paper on the autistic four-year-old girl I'd observed in a field placement contained more description than data; I was clearly more intrigued by her as a character than by the details of her diagnosis. By senior year, in my Cognitive Issues seminar, I was studying the psychology of language, writing papers about prototype theory and metaphorical thinking. I was testing my "right to write," too—taking a feature journalism class at the University of Pennsylvania, interning at *Philadelphia Magazine*, and publishing a bi-weekly editorial column in the *Bryn Mawr-Haverford Bi-College News*. And then one day in senior seminar, Professor Clark McCauley surprised me by saying he'd read my column. "Good work," he said casually, kindly. "You're going to make a living writing one day." This essay, written thirty years later, is just one fragment of my gratitude for the encouragement I heard—still hear—in my professor's words.

* * *

Saturday, April 22, 1922 clear, cool, brilliant
"PT said to Uncle Earnest, 'She is our best student'—I am elated, inspired —those murky misgivings and suicidal agonies retreat to deeper corners —though never do they entirely vanish. This is my clear ambition—honor by those I respect. More I demand still of course—honor from the world beyond academic doors—"

PT? I wondered as I read. I gasped out loud when I realized that the initials stood for President Thomas.

Elizabeth Mosier

I imagined Bryn Mawr's founding dean and second president, the legendary M. Carey Thomas, placing her hand upon Dorothy's shoulder, conferring her status—and sealing her fate. Though Dorothy had yet to choose her profession, she'd been chosen. She'd first been launched on a scholarly trajectory when her novelist mother, Anna Robeson Burr, suggested a career in archaeology; she'd gained momentum when she declared a double major in Classical archaeology and Greek. Now, with the president's endorsement and high praise from professors Rhys Carpenter and Mary Swindler, she set her sights on winning Bryn Mawr's European Fellowship—a prize that would cover a year of study in Greece, where she would begin the work that defined her life.

And yet, those archive boxes full of Dorothy's college diaries tell another story: that the work that fills our days is not always what we're remembered for.

* * *

The students in the Creative Writing Program at Bryn Mawr are smart, talented, and well trained to critically examine themes in literature—but they don't all share the "literary temperament." Some of the best writers I've taught are math and physics majors who learn, alongside English majors pursuing minors in creative writing, to think as writers—to understand and apply literary technique to produce a desired effect on the page.

At the end of the fall semester, we are talking about different kinds of story endings, including resonant images like James Joyce's "snow falling faintly through the universe" at the end of "The Dead." I tell my students that stories don't need to resolve neatly to be meaningful. If the writer has done her work with scene and exposition and sensory detail, the reader will feel that what has happened in the story mattered—in other words, that the depicted events have brought about a transformation that opens the story instead of tying it up.

Later, at my writing desk, I shuffle through several possible endings to Dorothy's narrative, drawing from the descriptions in her diary. Should I choose the Elizabethan festival of May Day, one of Bryn Mawr's most beloved traditions? Or Commencement, the academic year's culminating event? Or maybe Dorothy's chance reunion with her math professor, Agnes Scott, while out walking on April 8, 1923?

This last picture is almost too perfect. Dorothy describes how Miss Scott, one of M. Carey Thomas's first hires and true stars, contradicts the idea of the "scientific personality" by warmly greeting her former student "who deserted mathematics" and giving

28

her a bouquet of pansies picked from her own garden. "Just so you do one thing thoroughly, that's all that matters," Dr. Scott says to her. Dorothy, seemingly as surprised and touched as I am by her words, asks herself in her diary, "Was I wrong to leave the influence of such a spirit?"

Chronologically, this entry is nearer to the end of Dorothy's college years than the ending I have in mind for this essay. It also makes a point, perhaps too neatly, that there can be no definite resolution to Dorothy's dilemma. In this same passage—one week after winning the European Fellowship and being feted by professors and classmates and family—she is dismayed to hear that Rhys Carpenter (a name I associate with the modern, multi-million dollar addition to Bryn Mawr's art history and archaeology library) has described Dorothy's "heart's desire" as archaeology. She writes, "I almost want to scream 'No, no, no,'; to write and only to write and if not that—to create, be it but buttons!"

By this point in the story, Dorothy's character has been sufficiently illuminated; her "clear ambition—honor by those I respect" has been fulfilled. And so I choose to end instead with an image of Dorothy from an evening three weeks earlier, watching the windows of the president's office from her room in Pembroke Hall, as she awaits word of her brilliant future.

Thursday, March 15, 1923 clear, cold, brilliant
"This week has been a worse strain than the war zone—and then I was watching for Death! But the slow tightening of the web that draws me inescapably to the centre—ie: tonight when finally, undeniably, I shall know about the European Fellowship. After 4 years of doubt, it comes as a high culmination, particularly by so much drama..."
Later
8:00 pm The lights in Taylor make me uncommon nervous...
10:30 In an hour, it is about helpless!
10:50 All over! The letter, secured by adhesive tape, lies under the covers —and here's for a good sleep! So quiet a night for all these years! I rather hate to have it go!"

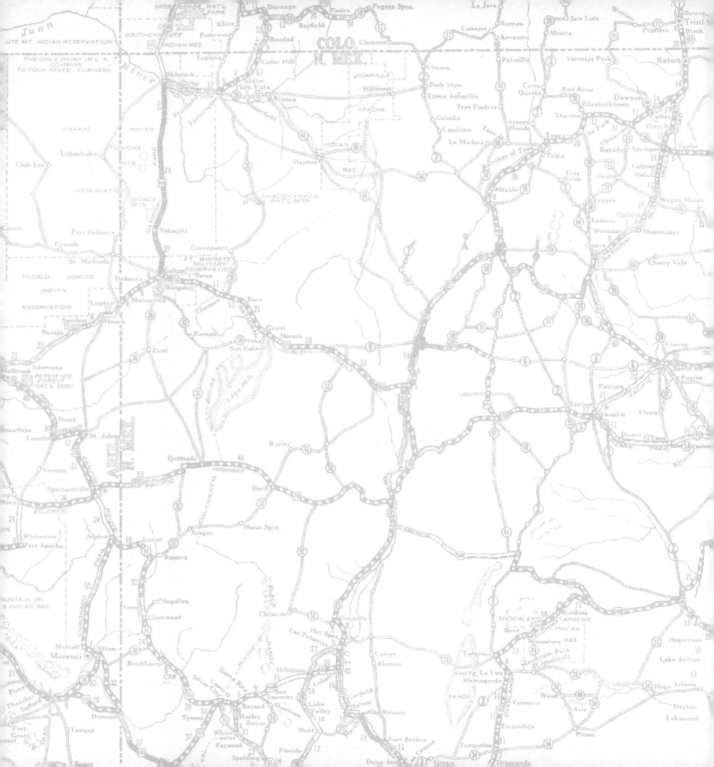

The Pit and the Page

When I talk about my volunteer work at the Independence National Historical Park Archeology Laboratory in Philadelphia, people often ask me if I've taken anything. Apparently, many people would pocket a sherd of broken glass or pottery as a souvenir if given half a chance. But these fragments of colonial history don't tempt me. They seem sacred, imbued with other people's stories. Besides, there are too many pieces for any one piece to be precious. I only have to enter the lab's storeroom and stand amid the rows of floor-to-ceiling shelves stacked with cartons (more than a million artifacts hauled up from a mile-square block of backyard privy pits) to feel the weight of history. Two sites—one named for George Washington's President's House that once stood at Sixth and Market, the other for the National Constitution Center that now stands on the vast lawn across the street—have yielded more treasures than the dig at Colonial Williamsburg. It will take ten years to process it all.

Today's assignment—brushing diluted adhesive across tiny field specimen numbers to seal the numbers inked onto hundreds of sherds—is Zen-like in its tedium. Hours pass, marked by the transfer of pieces, one by one, from mesh tray to aluminum, as the empty baker's rack is slowly filled. My time to think, I tell my friends. But really, I love the work because it requires just enough focus so that I can't think. I can't think about my mother, who is dying slowly and furiously. My grief is an unpacked box of sharp pieces stacked in a dark storeroom, while I lug around a catalogue of unfinished business.

This is my break from that.

* * *

At my mother's memory care community in Phoenix, I look out across the parking lot and see a cinderblock fence and, beyond it, the dull taupe houses made of chicken wire and stucco. My mother sees a timeline of her accomplishments—years bundled into numbered lots dotting the desert, constellations of housing developments named Saddleback Homes, The Meadow, Scottsdale Vista, Heritage Village, Mountainside Estates. There is no convincing her that these aren't her houses, the three-dimensional evidence of her long career in real estate.

"That's what I have to look at while I'm locked up in this prison," she says, gesturing to the space surrounding the gazebo where we sit. "Do you know how awful it is to be here when I used to be there?"

Her arm hangs in the air for a moment, as loose as a marionette's. Lately, her movements seem detached from her intentions, inspired instead by her body's memory. I feel that way, too—disconnected—sitting in this ridiculous gazebo in the center of a burnt-grass courtyard a few days before Christmas. I am performing, directing myself from a seat somewhere in the audience. I desperately don't want to be here, but this is what it's come to.

"A man from the state came yesterday. He says I don't belong here," she says.

"Would you like to open your presents?" I ask.

"You're not even listening to me," she says.

"I am listening."

"I'm going to kill myself."

Suicide has always been her backup plan, first voiced when I was ten years old, a child with her ear pressed against the hollow bedroom door while she sobbed into her pillow about a hairbrush she couldn't find and about ending her life. Even then, I knew that her complaint—"I have nothing! You kids take everything!"—was the screw-top cap on the deep jar of her grief. I sensed, too, that her dire plan would soon be abandoned, just like the weight-loss diets and new enthusiasms (extrasensory perception, horoscope, Phoenix Suns basketball, genealogy) and unopened patterns for child-sized clothes I recently found in the drawers of the old baby dresser in the back of her closet. For years, I listened at that locked door, one hand on the brass knob, reassured by her sobbing because it meant she was not dead.

"You don't mean that," I say.

She has lived to see seventy-five, only to lose her memory.

* * *

I began volunteering at the archaeology lab after taking a leave from teaching creative writing. My mother's dementia had reached a crisis, and I needed time: to rescue Dad, to move Mom into memory care, to prepare their house for sale. Like any teacher, I feared shortchanging my students—though it was more likely that I'd give my best self to my students and bicker with my brothers about what we should do to keep our parents safe. I anticipated a slow leak of my patience, the airbag between who I am and who I would become during the long, sad ordeal. And so, for the first time, I declined invitations to a season of Young Writers Day presentations at local elementary schools, and asked a colleague to take over my college course. Volunteering at the lab was a commitment I believed I could honor, since I'd be able to withdraw when my family needed me.

I'd first visited the President's House site just after the Independence National Historical Park archaeologists uncovered the foundation wall of the so-called "Philadelphia White House," including Washington's slaves' quarters. Just beneath the modern entrance to the glass house containing the Liberty Bell, there once lived Oney Judge, Moll, Austin, Hercules, Richmond, Giles, Paris, Christopher Sheels, and Joe Richardson.

Head archaeologist Jed Levin stood in the pit in his hard hat and told me how five long weeks of effort had yielded nothing but rubble and fill. And then he'd found the 1833 U.S. penny—"an omen," he said—placed by a mason to mark the boundary between the nineteenth-century storefront built that year and the colonial townhouse that lay below. For Jed, it was a career-making discovery, one that twined his life's purpose with his years of practiced skill. "This foundation isn't just bricks and mortar," he said, and I felt goosebumps rise along my arm. "It's a tangible link to the people who lived in this house, and a link between the enslaved and the free."

I was hooked. What writer doesn't understand the urge to look for truth beneath the surface, or the desire to tell the untold story? And what middle-aged teacher doesn't sometimes lament the energy she's expended on students, which might have been harnessed for her own discoveries? My mother's memory loss haunted me, warning me to make something tangible to account for my life. But though I'd cleared my desk of student work, I was too distraught and distracted to write. Processing artifacts from the President's House dig was a way of contributing to a bigger, more important story than mine.

By the time I was able to join the Thursday crew of graduate students and retirees, the staff had already completed work at that site. The ground had been filled in and grass-seeded; meanwhile, the city argued over the plan for a memorial that would reflect the complex truth about Washington and the nine enslaved Africans. And so my supervisor, Deborah Miller, set me to work washing the colonial dishes of the German, French, Irish, and free African Americans who'd lived in the dense block of rowhouses that had been cleared to give Bicentennial visitors a nicer view of Independence Hall.

I was disappointed, but still I signed on. After all, I was seeking solace, not story material. Four years later, I haven't missed a shift.

* * *

"I'm so bored," Mom says. "There's nothing to do here."

The activities calendar, offering Sittercise and Library Outing and Puzzles & Games and Art Class among other activities the staff says she enjoys, is posted on my refrigerator at home. In her room, a pile of unread *New Yorker*s my brother sent rests atop her wooden wardrobe. Blank crossword puzzles that some thoughtful person has clipped for her from the newspaper are stuffed into her dresser drawer. As far as I can see, her routine here is the same as it was in the house we had to sell to afford her care: pacing, watching television, picking fights. But we have ruined her life by putting her away in this place where she can't drive, can't hit our father, can't hang her broker's shingle and re-sell all those homes.

Last Christmas, I gave her a journal called *The Story of Your Life*, hoping its nostalgic leading questions—*Write about your best birthday*, *Describe your favorite pet*, *Did you have a secret hiding place as a child?*—would take her to the Indiana childhood she remembers fondly and vividly. In Art Class, she's filled a stack of pages with watercolor pictures featuring the family barn. I had hoped she might fill the journal with words that recall a happier life, but the book's spine is unbroken and its pages are unmarked.

"Where's your father?" she asks.

"He had a doctor's appointment," I say.

It's a lie, but here, lying is a strategy. And besides, it's what comes to mind whenever I think of our father, now: the blood bruises spotting his back, his broken thumb set in plaster, his arm immobilized by a sling. Defensive wounds, Dr. Cohen said, when she signed the letter that declared Mom a danger to herself and to others. Dr. Cohen is my hero. She saw and signed and legally documented what it's hard for others to believe: my father loves my mother so much that he risked his life defending her wish to continue living at home.

"That's a lie," Mom says. "He's got a lady friend."

"He does not have a lady friend," I say. Against professional advice, against logic, against my own will, I am arguing with her.

"He brought her here," she says. "Took her around and showed her off right under my nose."

"That's crazy," I say, a poor choice of words because they are true. I take a deep breath and try again. "Dad loves you. He's still your husband. He just couldn't visit today."

"Where's your father?" she asks again.

"He had a doctor's appointment," I say.

"That's a lie," Mom says.

I have never been good at lying.

I've discovered, through trial and mostly error while telling this unfolding story, that caring for a sick parent is like nursing a child: everyone has an opinion about how it should be done. By "everyone" I mean family, but also doctors, social workers, legislators, insurers, neighbors, colleagues, columnists, novelists, friends with sane parents, friends with long-dead parents, friends without children and not sandwiched as I am between needy kids and needier parents. Like the elder care advocates who have overrun Arizona, everyone talks about options, while somehow making clear that the only sanctioned choice for me—for any daughter—is to care for my mother in my home. To embrace the opportunity to give back what I have received from her. But I only need to remember my father's injuries to know why that's impossible.

Part of my inheritance is genetic, possibly latent, testable but inconclusively so. I collected the rest when I spent a week in my childhood home, cleaning up the chaos Alzheimer's disease has made of our family's life. Like an archaeologist, I have counted and catalogued and cartoned our history, hoping to make sense of the few sad relics I didn't sell or give to charity or bury in the dumpster behind the First Baptist Church.

* * *

I bring no skill but nearsightedness to the work of archaeology, and am regularly rewarded with writer-geek discoveries: the stub of a charcoal pencil, the intact lens from a pair of round eyeglasses, a bit of nineteenth-century newsprint stuck to a pottery bowl. But most days at the lab are more mundane. I label pieces of broken bottles—many of them the size of my pinky nail—using black or white ink applied with a nib pen. Or I dismantle bottles we've spent weeks mending with masking tape, and then catalogue the pieces by vessel number in the lab's database.

Urban archaeology is ethnography, staff archaeologist Willie Hoffman explained when I first began. The point of our work is not to preserve or display these artifacts, but to learn about the people who used them: their socioeconomic classes and customs, eating habits, manufacturing and trading patterns. Working alongside the archaeologists, learning their vocabulary and practicing their peculiar methods, I've come to see our jobs as similar. Writing is something like building a bottle from the base up using broken glass scattered on a table, glittering and inscrutable. And then taking it apart again to slowly fashion a story from the findings.

* * *

"This one's peanut brittle," I say, tearing through the wrapping paper to reveal the box of candy I brought to Mom from See's Candies at the mall. "Let's open it now, so you can share it with me."

"That's nice," she says, as she lifts the lid and fishes out the largest sherd. "It's my favorite."

"Mine, too," I say. "By coincidence."

She laughs, I laugh, and this is the moment I hold on to, the anecdote I will offer my father later, as evidence that things aren't as hopeless as they seem, and that it might be safe for him to visit soon. The day is warm for December in Phoenix, and the afternoon sun casts a flattering, soft, sideways light. Back in Philadelphia, my husband and daughters are trimming our tree, drinking cocoa, texting me funny messages to remind me of my other, parallel life.

Then Mom says, "He says I don't belong here." Meaning, of course, the Man from the State. He is her newfound deity.

"Hmm," I say, looking away.

"You don't believe me," she says, and when I look at her, look full into her face, I notice that her eyes seem unsecured. They roll strangely in their sockets, like a ball-bearing game, searching for their groove. "Your father has a lady friend. He had the nerve to bring her here."

"Nope," I say.

"I guess that's what happens to wives when they stop making money," she says. "They get put away."

"You probably saw Dad with someone who works here," I say. "He came by to bring you a new pair of Keds." Now I'm not only arguing, I'm lying with flourish. In fact, I bought and delivered the shoes myself when I visited at Thanksgiving. I dropped them off at the front office and fled when I saw my mother pacing the courtyard mechanically, wearing a ratty sweater and an angry scowl on her face.

"These shoes have ten more miles on them," she says, looking down at her old sneakers, at the white cotton sock pushing through the canvas where it's split across the top.

She will never wear the new shoes or the nicer sweater I sent her. She is, after all, the same woman who trashed a freezer full of casseroles I made for her while my father was in the hospital. It's possible she can't remember that these unfamiliar things are gifts.

I imagine handing her a wrapped box containing her old teddy bear, which she brought back from Indiana after her mother died. Back then, his arm was missing and one glass eye had been switched for a leather button, rendering the bear odd and half-blind. My mother had always planned to fix him, but he looked much the same when I found him thirty years later, on the top shelf in the hall closet. Considering Mom's other cast-off plans, which I'd unearthed during my dismal excavation of our family home, the bear's bad condition was distressing and not at all a surprise.

But in my daydream, I have done it. I have repaired him. I have gently bathed and combed his matted fur until his dreads fell loose and shone. I have made a small incision in his backside, vacuumed out his crumbled sawdust stuffing, and carefully replaced it with mold-resistant poly-fil. On his front left side, where his heart would be, I have tucked a sachet of dried lavender, and sutured him closed with invisible thread. I have restored his charm with matching round glass eyes, ordered online. I have consulted a specialist, my mother-in-law, an expert quilter who has carefully reattached his poor ragged arm.

I have wrapped him up with my childish wish in bright tissue paper and brought him to my mother, to reopen.

"What is it?" I imagine her saying, as she lifts her old bear from his box.

"Your teddy bear," I say.

She turns the bear over, inspecting his seams. "Sweetumpuss," she says. I had forgotten his name.

"I cleaned him up a bit," I say. "I re-attached his arm. Remember? You always wanted to do that."

"You took him," she says, and the familiar shape of gloom changes her face. "You take everything."

"I'm sorry," I say.

End scene.

It's true. I took the teddy bear, intending to repair and return him to Mom, but that was years ago now. The bear still rests on a shelf in my office, waiting for—what? Her death? Enough time to pass to diffuse its symbolic power?

I only wish I could fix it. Wishing, like lying, is a strategy. Storytelling is how I survived a childhood shaped by her sorrow, and how I moved a mountain of objects and heirlooms from my family's home without being crushed by grief.

* * *

Wandering through the antiques mall in Charlottesville, Virginia, during spring break, I stopped at one vendor's stand that was set up like a kitchen pantry, a nostalgic display of tin spice cans and rusty wire whisks and homespun kitsch of the Old South. Some of it was sadly similar to items I'd too recently let go of while preparing my childhood home for quick sale. I was still in mourning for my family's heirlooms; I'd barely had time to process what I'd been through. Perusing the carefully cased treasures inside the cool, quiet, funereal mall —quilts and tea sets and framed photos of someone else's ancestors—I was not exactly in a collecting mood.

And then, in a dusty breakfront cabinet, I found a set of blue Willow Ware. Deborah Miller had taught me to recognize the pattern by its geometric border design and its trio of figures crossing a bridge. "The three dudes," Debbie called them, with the affection of a material culture scholar who's handled thousands of broken pieces of eighteenth-century ceramics. But unlike most of the china I washed and labeled and repaired at the lab, these dishes were entirely, inexplicably intact.

I like working with Willow Ware because its narrative offers clues to aid its repair. Bottles come in distinctive shades of greens and browns, redware hints at matches with its swirling yellow slip, but only Willow Ware offers a pictorial legend: the story, told clockwise, of the Mandarin's daughter and her servant lover. Pursued by her father's chosen suitor, they escape across the bridge to a gardener's cottage, then by boat to an island, where the lover is killed and the daughter dies in a fire. They are transformed into immortal doves, surveying their own lives from the heavens, always positioned at twelve o'clock. Knowing the whole story helps me to find the missing pieces in the pile on the table and put the dishes together again.

That discovery—not a mason's penny, but a metaphor—signaled my own breakthrough. Already, my mother had forgotten my children; I knew that someday, she would forget me, too. Alone late at night in my childhood home, sorting through the flotsam of my family's history, I thought I knew how that story would end. But that day in the antiques mall, the Willow Ware reminded me of what every writer knows: you can't know the shape of a narrative until you reach the end of the draft.

I've worked at the lab long enough to know that what I don't know about archaeology is as vast as the storage room where the artifacts from The President's House and National Constitution Center digs are boxed up and shelved, alongside heavy cartons of sample soil. Long enough, too, to see that many of these broken things we work on day after day eventually become whole. I understand now that this slow, careful work—like grieving— is essential to the long process of repair.

* * *

In Mom's medical file, her neurologist narrates the progression of her symptoms, a grim path of "impressions" of a disease that can only be definitively diagnosed after death. *She is mostly oriented to time and place, intact to person. Memory is impaired for short-term but intact for long-term . . . She is partially oriented to time and mostly intact for place and is intact to person . . . She is mostly disoriented to time and place and is intact to person.*

I have added more recent impressions, taken as I observed Mom's art class when I visited at Thanksgiving:

At the front of the room is the still life the residents are to paint today: a fern, a few leaves, and a small pumpkin, backed by a Japanese screen. Mom paints, instead, a picture of the red barn in winter. When she's finished, she turns and sees you sitting in the corner of the room. She does not know who you are. You call her by name, you approach and admire her work, you caption her paintings with personal pronouns, you stand next to her offering the sensory clues of your face, your voice, your hand placed gently on her arm. "Is this your daughter?" asks a resident next to her, the lady in the pink velour tracksuit. "Yes," you say. Your mother says, "No."

There is no other way to say it. I felt erased.

And then I am mysteriously recalled. Today, she knows I am her daughter, sitting in a gazebo at a memory care center in Phoenix just before Christmas. She is, as the neurologist says, intact to person, place, and time. But the sad fact is, I'm not really there. I am still sitting at a table in her art class a month ago, my pen moving across the pages of my journal, beginning this essay.

"Where's your father?" Mom asks. "Why doesn't he come?"

"I don't know," I say. "But I'm here."

"I don't belong here," she says. "I'm going to kill myself."

"You don't mean that," I say, and kiss her dry forehead. "I love you. It's time for me to go."

"You don't even care," she says.

I rise and walk across the yard to the exit, repeating a mantra in my head: *she doesn't mean to she doesn't mean to she doesn't mean to.* At the gate that leads to the parking lot, I stop. The gate is locked, and I have forgotten the code. I always forget the code.

"Where are you going?" Mom calls out.

"Home," I say, thinking of my husband and daughters, our cedar-shingled Victorian house glittering with colored lights and iced with fallen snow. Too pretty a picture to be my life, and yet, miraculously, it is the life I've made.

"I don't want to die here," she says.

I look through the bars across the parking lot, to the familiar neighborhood of stucco homes. Say she did sell them. She might have sold them. I'm baffled by the gridded, sprawling city that lies beyond this gate, meticulously planned and utterly random. Why here, and not there? My mother has spent her life in these houses, all of them identically clean and tastefully staged. I raised myself elsewhere, and now I'm going home.

My cell phone buzzes in my pocket with a text from my brother, who's taken my place in the gazebo next to Mom. He sends me the code. I punch the numbers into the keypad and push open the gate.

"See you next time," I say, once I'm safely on the other side.

"This is the last time you'll see me," she says.

"See you next time," I say again.

I've stayed too long.

I had hoped to drive through our old neighborhood on the way to the airport, but now I have to take the highway so I won't miss my flight. I drive fast, remembering the icons of my childhood. I've keyed the map of my hometown for my daughters with stories of mishaps and tragedies, as if disaster defined the place. The citrus orchard (now an empty dirt lot) at 3rd Avenue and Northern, where a bunch of kids I knew were busted at an all-night party. The pawn shop on Central Avenue, where a man took a chainsaw from the shelf and tried to cut off his own head. My high school, where a gun-owning boy once tagged my name on the front wall. Next door, the Phoenix Indian School, where reservation kids were stripped of their tribal clothing and drilled in Anglo customs. The Hotel Clarendon, where an *Arizona Republic* reporter was blown up in his car for reporting on the mob. The St. Vincent DePaul Thrift Store, where my childhood writing desk is for sale. The now-empty house at Third Avenue and Glendale, where my family once lived.

When my family moved here, in 1964, the desert was vast, a blank canvas. Flying into the valley at night, the city lights appeared suddenly out of the darkness, and every single time it surprised me. Back then, there were still places where bobcats and rattlesnakes and chuckwallas lived, still places where teenagers could tap a keg undetected, still plenty of places to hide. But Phoenix, for me, has irrevocably changed. Now there are freeways stretching out across the desert, erasing the old landmarks, speeding me into the future, and I don't know where I am.

* * *

There's a meditative aspect to the tasks of archaeology: washing, labeling, and mending artifacts; counting and bagging animal bones; sorting through residuals sifted from dirt that's been washed through a one-eighth-inch mesh screen.

The trick to this last task, called "picking," is to tackle no more than a quarter-sized pile at a time. First, you scrape the gravel across the tray with a tongue depressor; next, with a tweezer, you separate the contents by type: brick, mortar, bone, charcoal, flora (seeds), metal, miscellanea (buttons, beads, straight pins, teeth), insects, and oyster shell. It took many hours of practice before I knew what I was seeing: a splinter of cream-colored egg shell, a transparent fish scale, the fibrous backside of what looked at first like charcoal but was really a bit of burnt bone.

Wash, sort, label, mend, and catalogue. At the lab, I work through the mountain one molehill at a time. As I work, I think about life's lost objects and found wisdom, about the mysterious ways memory serves and finally fails us, about the fragments that float to the surface or fall through the screen. I think about how the words we choose to tell a story enclose and connect our unfinished business and unsettled feelings just as tangibly as a building's bricks and mortar do. The art is in the process, whether the story's being told in the pit or on the page.

* * *

By now, the Thursday archaeology lab volunteers are like family to me, with their set roles, stubborn habits, and particular talents. Randy, a retired librarian, leans over a table full of broken bottles he's been trying to rebuild for weeks. Carolyn, a retired physical therapist, inks black numbers onto pottery with her personal nib pen, cursing under her breath when a clot forms and smears. Dick, a retired Lutheran pastor, and his wife Nancy, a retired teacher, arrive after lunch to help wherever they're needed.

On such a day, when the room hums with library quiet, I can hear the ghosts of the past whispering through these recovered artifacts: the shattered Madeira glasses, the musket balls and curled shoe leather, the pharmaceutical bottle embossed with SWAIM'S VERMIPUGE (a quack cure for cholera), the rotten bicuspid, the gold wedding ring. *Let go*, I imagine these broken, discarded objects saying. *Everything, from the trivial to the treasured, finally ends up in the privy pit.* I find strange comfort in that sober message, which humbles and empowers any writer to seek the universal in the personal—to make meaning, which is the artifact of experience.

The Farmer's Guide Cook Book

My maternal grandmother's 1927 *Farmer's Guide Cook Book* is more than a book of old recipes. The scraps she pasted and pinned to and slipped between its pages—home remedies, magazine clippings, shopping lists, poems, a postcard, a program for a piano recital—are markers of social identity. As an artifact, her cookbook is a window into the practices and politics of a particular time, place, and people in American history, and a grease-splattered record of her life in Frankfort, Indiana.

Among the ephemera I find inside are three different recipes for homemade soap, one with a preamble that seems to date it to the Great Depression: "In these days of high prices for what we buy and low prices for what we sell, it behooves us to watch every penny and save what we can."

There's a poem from 1931, "Unchanged," by the sentimental and optimistic Edgar A. Guest. Also known as "The People's Poet," Guest appeared on a weekly Detroit radio show from 1931–42, and on television (NBC's *A Guest in Your Home*) in 1951. He was later mocked by Dorothy Parker (who wrote, "I'd rather flunk my Wasserman [antibody test for syphilis] test / than read the poetry of Edgar Guest") and by Lemony Snicket (who claims in *The Grim Grotto*, the eleventh book in *A Series of Unfortunate Events*, "every noble reader in the world agrees that [Guest] was a writer of limited skill, who wrote awkward, tedious poetry on hopelessly sentimental topics.").

On the back of a handwritten recipe for Never Fail Cake Icing is a bill for *The Pathfinder* (1894–1954), a precursor to *Time* that "prints the gist of the world's news in a nutshell." A sternly personal note in green ink is signed by editor George D. Mitchell: "I'm sure you realize this is long past due. Please send your remittance. You know you'd miss *The Pathfinder* terribly if you didn't have it." The magazine's circulation was one million in 1936, the year Mitchell retired (and my mother was born). I don't know why my grandparents let it lapse.

The same year Jack Kerouac coined the term "The Beat Generation," my grandmother clipped an article from the August, 1948, issue of *Country Gentleman*, a popular magazine for rural readers put out by Curtis Publishing Co. in Philadelphia. But was she interested in how to freeze corn or (on the reverse side) how to make an apron out of a pair of bandanas? With cotton fabric back in abundance after wartime shortages, articles like this one reminded women that their real work was in the kitchen. But what did bandanas mean to my grandmother? Were they simply the bright-colored rags that farmers and cowboys traditionally wore around their necks to wipe the sweat off their faces and keep dust out of their collars? Or did they evoke Rosie the Riveter, her famous red head wrap symbolizing her readiness for work that would bring the boys home?

It seems my grandmother once drove over two hours from Frankfort to Goshen, Indiana, to hear a recital given by the students of Noble Kreider, a composer whose works are catalogued in the New York Public Library. Composer Arthur Farwell praised him in the May 22, 1909, issue of *Musical America*, writing, "Kreider's music revealed also an imaginative quality of its own, which asserted itself with increasing strength in his more recently composed works, and indicated that here was a personality which was bound to find its way to individual expression." Despite this national acclaim, Noble Kreider made a career of teaching in Goshen, his hometown, and died there in 1959.

My grandmother's ambitions were manifest in my mother's blue-ribbon baking and masterful piano playing. But not one to waste a piece of paper, she used the back of the recital program to copy a recipe for Gooseberry Cobble.

From Scratch

RHUBARB PIE

Use 1 cupful rhubarb cut into ½-inch lengths, 1 cupful seeded raisins, 1 beaten egg, juice of 1 lemon, 1 cupful sugar, 2 tablespoonfuls butter, cinnamon, nutmeg and allspice to suit taste. Mix together well, place in unbaked rich pastry, sprinkle with flour, place cover and bake. This makes two small pies.

GOOD PIE CRUST

Sift together well 1 ½ cupfuls pastry flour, ½ teaspoonful baking powder and a little salt. Work into this with tips of fingers ⅔ cupful lard and then add enough ice water to make a soft dough. This will make enough dough for two pie shells or one covered pie.

I.

Let there be pie. Let me bring it, still warm, to my father on a white china plate. Let the storm door bump my bare heel as I step outside onto the porch, a slice of his favorite rhubarb pie in each hand, two forks tucked into yellow napkins. Let it be noon, three years back, August, cool. Let baskets of pink impatiens hang from the eaves, nesting new birds kicking soil from the sky. Let the air smell of season's end: scorched earth, creosote, fermenting fruit. Let oakleaf hydrangea shade this corner where he sits watching weather, waiting for the promised rain. Let a leafy hand reach out to touch his shoulder, hold him fast, as I set his plate down on the table draped in sea blue cloth. Let him smile. "Here," let me say, "I made this for you," and with this gift, let him see that he taught me how to hope when he made things by hand.

II.

When the rain comes, let us go. For once, let me act without permission or expert advice. Let us pack the car with ballast—canned food and bottled water and a battery-powered lamp—and head west with a half-tank of gas and no backup plan. As streets become rivers, as strong winds draw dark currents across the sky, let me navigate by the shimmering stars of his memory. When he says, "Home," let me know what he means: Eden of elm trees; Mother's wildflower garden behind the house; furry-bird bat found on the way to school; the Hoosier Pete's gas station his father built; brand-new brick library; forbidden pool hall; ancient Indian burial mounds; Pennsylvania Railroad trains pulling steam as they pass through to Richmond or Mackinaw City, Michigan; poor drowned boy pulled, blue and still, from the quarry; Homer Hinshaw's biplane in pieces in a field; pork & beans and cornbread and rhubarb pie from Wick's; Luther and Nellie planting phlox on the land they bought from Charley Owens near the end of their lives. Let me unfold his map, hand drawn in blue ballpoint and keyed all in CAPS. Let us find "Lynn, Indiana, Circa 1950," unchanged and intact.

III.

It's late, but let me try. Let me return to Lynn with my father's ashes, guided by the map he made for me from memory when I went to my grandpa's funeral. Let me circle the perimeter of the hometown he never revisited, trying to make sense of twenty-three years of decline. Let me find his house on Main Street, though its number is different and the shade tree is gone. Let me walk the path to Owens's farm, where I once picked my grandparents' phlox in a yard now barred by a NO TRESPASSING sign. Let me seek shelter from the sun in the deserted library, where a woman blows smoke at a computer screen playing *The Price is Right*. Cracked windows, vacant storefronts, a Main Street of disappeared shops with gaps like missing teeth: let me see Lynn as it really is, not how I wish it to be. In the cemetery where Luther and Nellie are buried by two coffin-shaped voids, let me kneel on dead grass and feel the anguish of the forsaken. Let me be stingy with what is left of him, spilling a tablespoon of ash where his headstone would be. Let me keep the rest.

IV.

Let August, then, be my season of grief. When rhubarb appears in the market made quaint by bushel baskets and fake wood floors, let me see this as a sign. Let me take these last-ditch, greening stalks to my kitchen, crank open windows and crack open my grandmother's 1927 cookbook published by *Farmer's Guide*. While, outside, humidity and hissing cicadas speak of a storm and its aftermath, of the flood and of the fire, of what was and what will be, let me find the old recipe for rhubarb pie. Let me honor my inheritance. Let my hands do what my heart cannot. Let me begin again.

In self-imposed exile from the internet, let me consult this family Bible, splattered with stains and stuffed with the ephemera of Depression-era rural Indiana. Granddaughter of farmers, daughter of a 4-H blue-ribbon baker, let me be awed by my ancestors' expertise in making soap, butchering and smoking meat, grinding sausage, separating grain from its hull. Let me be humbled, listening to a language I don't speak fluently:

"The morning before you wish to bake, take ⅔ cupful of sweet milk (morn-ing milk is best), and let come to a boil . . ."
"This recipe is for 250 pounds of meat . . ."
"Gather a peck of tomatoes . . ."
"This is a fine dish for washing or ironing day . . ."

Let me close my eyes and conjure my grandmother in her farmhouse kitchen, making food not as solace, but as fuel. Let me read the recipe out loud, evoke the poetry of history connecting me through this heirloom to those who came before me, to those who have

Elizabeth Mosier

gone. Let my coffee go cold, let my phone go unanswered, let work deadlines wait as I labor at grief. Let me make a rhubarb pie to mark this time of transformation: his death and my life, there and then and here and now.

V.

Before I falter, let me remember that a recipe is not a formula, but a guide. Let me improvise: replace lard with butter, use Pyrex pie plate in place of tin, guess 400 degrees for the oven temperature and 50 minutes' baking time. Let me learn to trust my senses. Let me pinch chilled butter and flour between my fingers without visual aid or adjective ("pea-sized" or "crumb") until, on my own authority, the mixture feels "right." Let me experiment: add ice water a few drops at a time, press and squeeze to form silken dough. Let me taste raw rhubarb and find it bitter, densely grained as sand, and good. Let me gather plant and fruits and egg and sugar cane, and mix these with spices measured "to (my) taste." Let me divide the dough and roll each half on my Formica countertop, until world-shaped and wafer-thin. Let one disc serve as basin and the other, firmament. Let it bake until the filling bubbles and the crust is golden brown and the kitchen smells of sweet and sour, joy and sorrow, and I am home again.

VI.

Let me learn, let me practice, let me make mistakes. Today, let me sit on the porch with my pie and a pile of his artifacts: *Caterpillar Earthmover Performance Handbook*, copper-colored name badge, gold-plated wristwatch marking forty years, skeleton key to a long-ago tractor. Let these salvaged objects be my salve. Let them bind mind to body, experience to insight, as I travel this circuitous route. Let me pack and unpack these memories so many times that my mind receives them like an old, worn baseball glove shaped for the blow. Let me recall how he flailed for days as fluid filled his lungs. "Home," he said. Inventor, protector, eternal optimist: let him rest. Let his daughter sit in his chair on home's threshold and put the severed parts together, create order from chaos,

48

make sense of this new world. Let pain become revelation as I draft and revise, remember and return.

VII.

And after, let there be brown fields on this journey, desert before the bounty. Let there be rest stops along the way, where a tattooed, leather-clad motorcyclist lurks. Let me speak to this bandana-clad man, a Caterpillar mechanic who knows the machines my father labored on. Let there be a bridge between me and the vast expanse of what I don't know. Let there be softness, surrender, the absence of fear. Let me be wrong. Let me be surprised. Let there be kindness, and let it spread haphazardly, like the phlox that replants itself in a new place in my yard every year. Let me walk Main Street in Lynn once again, and let the answers I'm looking for be what I don't find. Let me sit at the counter at Mrs. Wick's and order a slice of rhubarb pie. Let me open my notebook and begin: "When he says home, let me know what he means." Let there be light in this darkness. Let me write to make hope visible, to keep faith with the amazing.

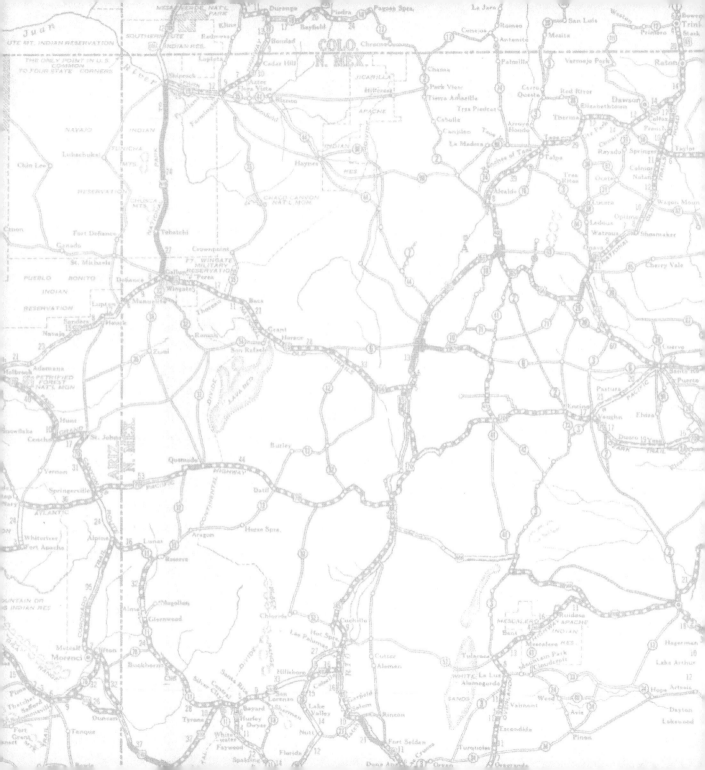

The Social
Life of Maps

My husband and I drove to the lecture at Stenton without looking at a map, our route plotted by GPS. The irony of a disembodied voice directing us to a lecture on "The Social Life of Maps in 18th-century America" wasn't lost on me. Nor was the novelty of navigating by satellite to the 1730 home of James Logan, secretary to William Penn and (among his many offices) colonial mayor of Philadelphia. I grew up using printed maps. If you're reading this essay in printed form, you probably did, too.

There is more to a map than topography, and the sold-out Saturday afternoon talk by Martin Brückner, a professor of English and associate director of the Center for Material Culture Studies at the University of Delaware, offers proof. Fifty-plus people—academics and archaeologists, students and armchair geographers—crowd Stenton's stone carriage house to discuss the rise of maps in popular culture in early America. Using images from the exhibit he curated at The Winterthur Museum in Winterthur, Delaware, Dr. Brückner traced maps from production to purchase to public display and personal use, as they became fashionable objects in the period before and after the Revolutionary War.

Maps introduced North America to European explorers and colonists, confirmed the colonies' independence, and documented the expansion of the United States. Literally and figuratively, maps shaped our country's image. But in the Age of Reason, function followed form; though Henry Popple's 1733 *A Map of the British Empire in America* was criticized for inaccuracy, Benjamin Franklin bought three copies, for his home and to hang in the Pennsylvania State House, as wall cover intended to assert authority and impress foreign diplomats.

In the eighteenth century, maps were everywhere: advertised with luxury goods in catalogues and with necessities in the newspaper; displayed in taverns and town halls and high-traffic areas in private homes; printed on parlor screens and ceramics and neckties —"cartifacts" serving no cartographic purpose. If political conflict built the market for maps, the cartouche—or decorative map title—refined it, adding beauty to the criteria for determining a map's value. The brisk business in maps for navigating and decorating redefined what constituted their usefulness, in material and social terms. Owning a map meant economic status, educational achievement, and national identity; showing a map showed you belonged.

This is the "performative function" of maps, to create reality by plotting it. Cartographers, writers, citizens: our histories derive from this belief in the concept of surveyable space.

My home state, Arizona, was settled with land status maps. My parents' careers— Dad's selling earthmoving equipment, Mom's selling houses—were enabled by accurate and alluring cartography. My grandparents' farm acreage in Indiana was established by boundary survey. I descend from soldiers rewarded for service in the 1811 Battle of Tippecanoe with frontier land John Melish encompassed in his 1816 *Map of the United States with the Contiguous British and Spanish Possessions*, regarded as the visual embodiment of Manifest Destiny. My German kin sailed to Philadelphia in 1728 on the *James Goodwill* and landed in the Perkiomen Valley, perhaps persuaded by the same map James Logan used: Thomas Holme's 1683 *A Mapp of Ye Improved Part of Pennsylvania in America Divided into Countyes, Townships and Lotts*.

A copy of Holme's map hangs in the house at Stenton today, on loan from Logan descendant Edward Middleton Drinker. Only temporarily, curator Laura Keim explains, as winter's stable temperature and humidity permit. Paper artifacts require careful climate control, and so the map is permanently on deposit with The Library Company of Philadelphia. This shared stewardship makes possible today's exhibit, which features other historic maps from Drinker's collection and treasures imported from Jonathan Cresswell's Philadelphia Print Shop, including a page of Georg Braun and Franz Hogenberg's *Civitates Orbis Terrarum*, an armchair traveler's compendium of bird's-eye views published in 1572. Brückner's expertise illuminates the display, fostering dialogue among colleagues and strangers. The event illustrates what Philadelphia's cultural institutions maintain: material culture and social life.

Lucky guests, we circulate through the gallery. When I get to the Holme map, I lean in to read it; like everyone else, I'm mentally walking the terrain, looking for emblems of my lived experience, mapping my personal geography. In the way that the past accrues to form identity, reading a map of a familiar place lets us find who we are in where we have been.

Recently, I took a walk with my daughters in Rittenhouse Square. Though I've keyed their map of Philadelphia with culture—art, theater, music, history—they wanted to see the apartments I rented in my twenties, data that's suddenly relevant as my older daughter prepares to graduate from college. As we walked, we mapped; my hidden history emerged in stories. I'm still studying Philadelphia, but thirty-five years after moving east from Phoenix, I'm surprised to find that I know this city better than I know my hometown.

Today, we use many tools to locate ourselves in society: geospatial analysis, political maps colored with symbolic red and blue, the Global Positioning System that simplifies geography by eliminating irrelevant details. While these maps provide an overview, they lack the inside stories of, say, the hand-drawn map of my father's hometown, the floor plan of the Indiana farmhouse where my mother was raised—just two of the many maps that brought me here. That is to say, home: a landscape mapped by memory; a place we eventually, with time, come to understand.

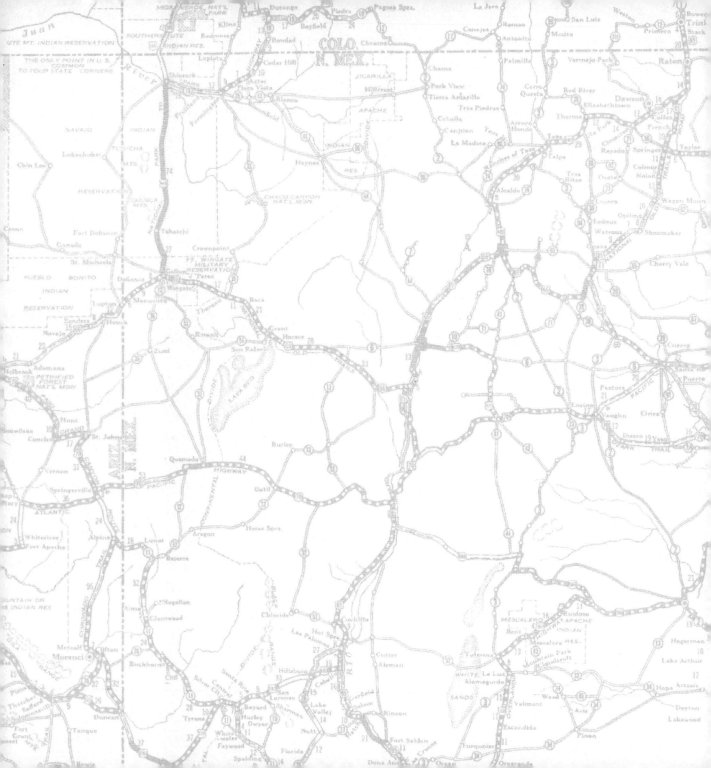

Memorial

It's high tourist season in Philadelphia, and so not at all unusual—if slightly unsettling—to find a man walking beside me on the regional rail platform clad in breeches, buckled shoes, and a tri-corner hat. He's commuting, as I am, to Independence National Historical Park, but he's costumed for interpreting history at the Visitors' Center, while I'm clad in privy-picker jeans and a black t-shirt for my volunteer work at the archaeology lab.

Like any city, Philadelphia has its versions: public and private, seen and unseen, drafted and revised. This summer morning, the two of us proceed down busy Market Street, parting at Sixth Street, the location of George Washington's residence and slaves' quarters from 1790–97. This complicated narrative—democracy framed upon the faulty foundation of slavery—first drew me to the site, when a team of archaeologists revealed the mortared stone walls of the "Philadelphia White House" and, in the process, disturbed the surface of a story last interpreted for the United States Bicentennial.

When I first visited the dig with my daughters, I couldn't help but read the emerging revision as a writer would. There, in the ground, was the visible footprint of the bow-windowed room that architectural historians say is the precedent to the modern-day Oval Office. Washington added it to the house for the purpose of meeting visitors at his level, not elevated and enthroned like a king. And there, five feet away, was the open-hearth kitchen where the enslaved man called Hercules cooked the president's meals.

One version of the story is shaped by this proximity: the symbol of democracy next to the brick and mortar evidence of slavery. Here, in this ironic setting, Hercules rises from plantation slave to celebrated chef, his talents and loyalty to Washington rewarded with unusual privileges. He makes an income from selling kitchen scraps, buys and wears fine clothing, strolls Philadelphia's abolitionist streets. Narrative tension is sustained by the dissonance between text (the appearance of liberty) and subtext (the reality of bondage) —and is resolved satisfyingly in March, 1797, when Hercules escapes.

Or so the story goes. Structurally, this version is as elegant as the portrait presumed to be of Hercules, painted by Washington's own portraitist, Gilbert Stuart. But portraiture is not a story. And that is the problem at the root of this narrative: a complete dramatic action is elusive when the protagonist isn't free to act. Or when the protagonist vanishes.

If this were fiction, the writer might attempt to open and deepen the draft by shifting narrative point of view. Seeing events through Hercules's eyes would compel the writer to develop him as a character, and not simply present him as an ironic figure in Washington's conflicted tale.

But this is history, and only facts can free the narrative from the limits imposed by its frame. In fact, the age and provenance of the famous portrait isn't fixed. The tall toque Hercules wears is a style that wasn't popular until later, in the early nineteenth century; Stuart scholars don't acknowledge the painting as part of the artist's body of work. And a recent discovery by Mt. Vernon research historian Mary V. Thompson not only recasts the story's climax, but also offers an ending that opens into Hercules's more probable future.

In the Mt. Vernon farm report dated February 25, 1797, Hercules is listed as "absconded for four days," meaning he fled to Philadelphia, not from it (as Washington later wrote in a letter to his secretary, Tobias Lear). Meaning Washington's birthday (February 22) was the occasion for his flight. As Washington hosted dignitaries in Philadelphia, the culinary artist supposedly valued for his skill and loyalty had in fact been at Mt. Vernon, assigned to the hard labor of digging clay for bricks—and, it turns out, plotting his escape.

The portrait of Hercules—which journeyed to aristocratic residences in Paris, France, and Gloucestershire, England, before reaching its current home in Spain's Museo Thyssen-Bornemisza—could have been painted by someone other than Stuart, after Hercules fled to Europe and joined the household of a British diplomat.

As Independence National Historical Park archaeologist Jed Levin explained to me when I first signed on to the long project of processing artifacts, archaeological research illuminates what's uncovered at the dig. Though the ground at the President's House site is now covered, the search for hidden stories continues.

* * *

In the end, it didn't surprise me that the "interpretive text" for the President's House memorial took longer to construct than the ghost structure built at the site to enclose this monumental story.

The first draft, briefly on display at the Independence Visitor Center, elicited conflicting reviews (too concerned with slavery, not concerned enough with slavery, dominated by well-known figures like Washington and Adams) and rare consensus that the long-awaited memorial was "unimaginative." Writing crafted by committee is often mediocre, in part because the process of compromise moves vivid, often opposing, views toward the duller middle. And this particular project is constrained by a marketing agenda that's separate from its historical one. You sense the rush to reassure visitors with a balanced presentation that seeks to "brand" Philadelphia even as it liberates the stories of Washington's nine slaves: Moll, Austin, Richmond, Giles, Paris, Christopher Sheels, Joe Richardson, Oney Judge, and Hercules.

But there is judgment in any narrative, whether overtly stated or conveyed by framing, emphasis, and omission. As a writer, what I found most revealing in the draft was the persistent use of passive voice to tell the story of slavery: *History is lost* to these Africans, who *were kidnapped and transported to America* and *given new names* and *forced to learn a new language*. The agent is missing in these constructions—either unknown or (still) unacknowledged.

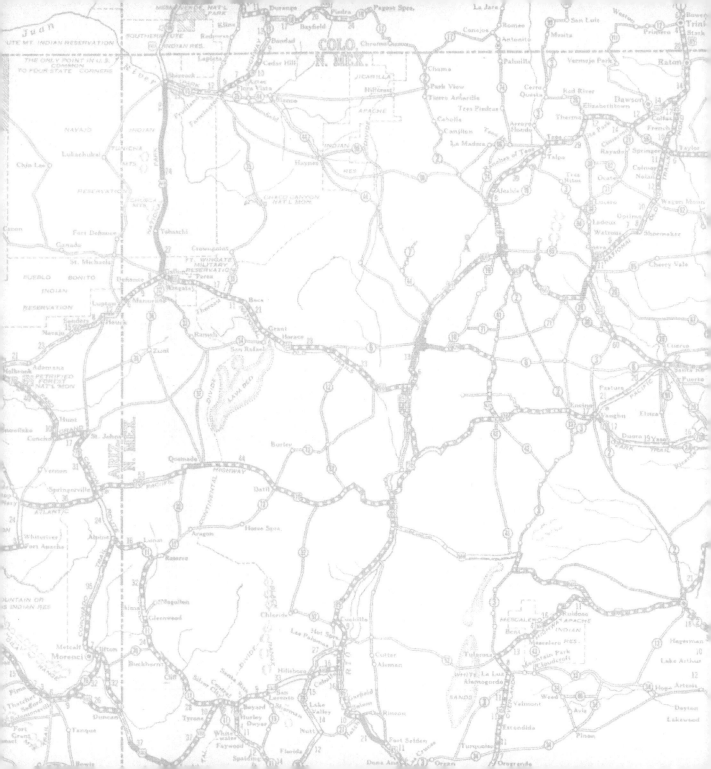

Love on a Plate

When our daughter moved into her first apartment last summer, I resisted the atavistic urge to set her up in wedding shower style, and gave her our chipped Crate & Barrel plates instead. Then I brought our wedding china up from the vintage IKEA cabinet in the basement for everyday use, breaking middle-class protocol to store or show off what we're rich enough to not need to use.

"Silver Ermine": the white-on-white Wedgwood pattern, with its floral ghost rim and platinum edge, is fairly plain though still too fancy for the casual hosts my husband Chris and I turned out to be. But bone china is strong and durable; by the season of our 30th anniversary, I wasn't afraid of breaking it. As I'd learned over seven years of working as an archaeological lab technician, true treasures bear the marks of use—especially plates, on which our daily sustenance and much of life's pleasure is served.

So, though this ceramics swap might look like a midlife promotion to finer dining, my motive was archaeological. Nearly a thousand hours of volunteering at the lab—washing and labeling a colonial neighborhood's glass fragments and ceramic sherds, mending its bottles and vessels and plates—has trained me to see broken things as material evidence: of social class, consumer patterns, cultural practices, politics, relationships. Though these days much of our stuff ends up in landfills instead of backyard privy pits, the things we risk losing by using them tell a truer story of how we live than the heirlooms we pack away for posterity.

What will our wedding china say about us?

An archaeologist would "read" our plates in their cultural context: post-Industrial Revolution American life, in which overproduction made china cheap enough for middle-class people to keep an extra set merely for meaning—the symbol of union, the ritual of the holiday dinner, the heirloom handed down. Our collection of twelve matching place settings bought at Wanamaker's (now Macy's) in Philadelphia speaks of the modern tradition of the department store bridal registry, started in 1924 at Chicago's Marshall Fields and still going strong when we married in 1985. That our plates remain unbroken today says something about our locational stability. We've lived most of our life together in the same house, a 1906 cedar-shingled Nantucket Victorian that more mobile neighbors in our small suburban tract of eight seem to view as a "starter home," but which—it's clear now, if it wasn't yet clear when we moved in—will be the first and last we own.

Then there is meaning to be found in the plates themselves. China production and patterns, like fashion and fabrics and technology, can be pinned to a particular place and time. Wedgwood bone china, which is refined to its characteristic translucence with humble cow bone ash that's added to white clay and a compound stone called pentunse, was first manufactured by Josiah Wedgwood II in 1812, in Staffordshire, Stoke-on-Trent, England. The company that Josiah's father built, by marketing expensive ornamental wares to the aristocracy and expensive useful products to the aspirocracy, was iconic in the 1980s wedding industrial complex that Chris and I tried our best to dodge.

But even I—a non-bridey bride who kept her name, cut her hair pixie-short, and wore a simple "tea-length" wedding dress scored wholesale by the fashion editor at the magazine where I worked—bought into tradition by choosing the Wedgwood brand. The pattern we picked is telling, too. "Silver Ermine" was produced from 1971–93, a timeline tracking my Baby Boomer cohort's coming of age and spanning the eras of hippie chic, Charles and Diana, and the "destination wedding." Our pattern's production life cycle coincided historically with a period when, according to the National Center for Health Statistics, the rising American divorce rate peaked (in 1981) and fell (in 1985), from 5.3 to 3.6 divorces per 1,000 people.

What were we thinking, getting married at a time when half of all marriages ended in divorce? For cultural context, my Bryn Mawr classmates were preparing for brilliant careers and PhDs, while I was making up a writing life as I went along. I never meant to marry—until, among the pre-med and "pre-money" Haverford men I dated (to use a verb that dates me), I met the one who wrote songs and played guitar in a band called "Victims of Entropy," whose hands were stained with oil paint and Plaster of Paris, whose dorm room smelled of linseed oil and possibility. Love is never simple, but simply put: Chris made things, and he saw and understood the life of meaning making that I envisioned for myself.

We were so young! I didn't understand how young, though, until the day last summer when, watching our daughter pack up our hand-me-down household items for her new apartment, I remembered myself at her age—asking Chris Mills to marry me. Her boyfriend at the time was a truly lovely man, who is smart and talented and handsome; the two were playing the long game within a contemporary collegiate culture that seems to view marriage as either unnecessary or the last item on a list of accolades. I was half-afraid she'd follow her parents' youthful example, and half-afraid she wouldn't.

My mother, who married my father when she was just shy of nineteen, worried about me, too; she (quite reasonably) feared I'd follow Chris as he pursued his ambitions, instead of pursuing my own. Yet it was she who urged us to register for china, despite our far more pressing needs (rent, our first word processor, tuition for my master's degree). She said, "You can't know at twenty-two what you'll want when you're thirty."

She was right. Not in the metaphorical terms that clever fine china manufacturers use to sell their wares—a couple's choice of china pattern as the blueprint for their married life —but rather, in terms of the fact-against-faith reality that best-laid plans often go awry. In fact, by the time I turned thirty, Chris and I had changed jobs, career plans, cities, houses, and our minds on the issue of having children. We no longer resembled the people who'd walked down the aisle. But I think we're still together today because, when we chose to marry, we chose to change together.

Our wedding china links us to history, and tells part of a bigger, broader story of human experience (and exclusion from experience) with the institution of marriage. But the smaller, more personal story—our lives with these plates—starts with evidence of ownership and use: the list of people we thanked for their wedding gifts; the Replacements, Ltd. receipt for eight "Silver Ermine" soup bowls purchased recently (because, as it turns out, we like soup); photos of three decades of holiday dinners featuring our china holding a heap of turkey and stuffing or a slice of chocolate birthday cake. And also, from now on, the Wedgwood plates stacked in the kitchen cabinet, sharing shelf space with vintage Deruta bowls and Picardie tumblers and Bennington Pottery coffee mugs. Our wedding china, earning symbolic value through daily circulation; becoming marked and therefore memorable.

My parents were married for sixty years, as were my in-laws. I admit that I used to view long-lasting marriages like theirs as uneventful, the way mobility researchers studying neighborhoods reveal their bias by asking why people move but not how they stay. Divorce, after all, is a story—one with inherent conflict, a perceived antagonist, a dramatic turning point, and a meaningful dénouement. Our good friends' stories of splitting up are punctuated with painful events, including wedding china being hurled to the floor or hauled off to a consignment shop. But a symbol isn't a story, and the unbroken marriage, like the intact plate, used to seem to me inscrutable.

Archaeology made me think differently. The way artifacts accrue meaning over time, the way history is layered in the privy pit, suggested a new way to interpret the phrase, to have and to hold. Our practices reveal our intentions, which is one reason we look back at what we've done to understand how we belong within a culture—how we resist and how we compromise.

If I consider stability, *staying*, as an analytic category and not merely as the absence of an event, then our wedding china indicates a commitment we've made to each other every day, on and on for thirty years. This symbol of a long-ago promise reveals the depth of our intimacy with each other and with the home we've made. And tracing the artifact back to its origins helps me to describe the cultural landscape in which our intentions—starting with our decision to marry—set us down the circuitous path that led us here: a week away from our thirty-first anniversary, our route changed by the choices we've made together.

At this point, there is no one on earth who knows Chris or me as well as we know each other. We have marked each other; we are each other's history. As the archaeological record reveals, there is the artifact and the interpretation, the symbol and the story, the deep meaning and the daily practice—and we all live in these two realms at once.

* * *

"The Thanksgiving plates," Chris said, when he opened the kitchen cupboard and discovered the wedding china I'd stacked there.

"We're celebrating," I told him, meaning any day without a crisis, which he understood. We've lived through the midlife pileup together—career disillusionment, financial stress, health problems, teenagers' troubles, parents' deaths—and we are giddy to still be here. Dining on our still-pristine plates feels like reclamation.

Once, at the archaeology lab, as I washed broken dishes and set them to dry on the wood-framed mesh screens, the sight of all those jumbled, broken belongings made me say out loud, "That was some party!" I hope that one day, our wedding china—with its inevitable chips, cracks, stains, tarnished edges, bases cross-hatched with scratches from diners' knives and forks—will tell our daughters the story of our long and happy marriage, and that they'll say the same of us.

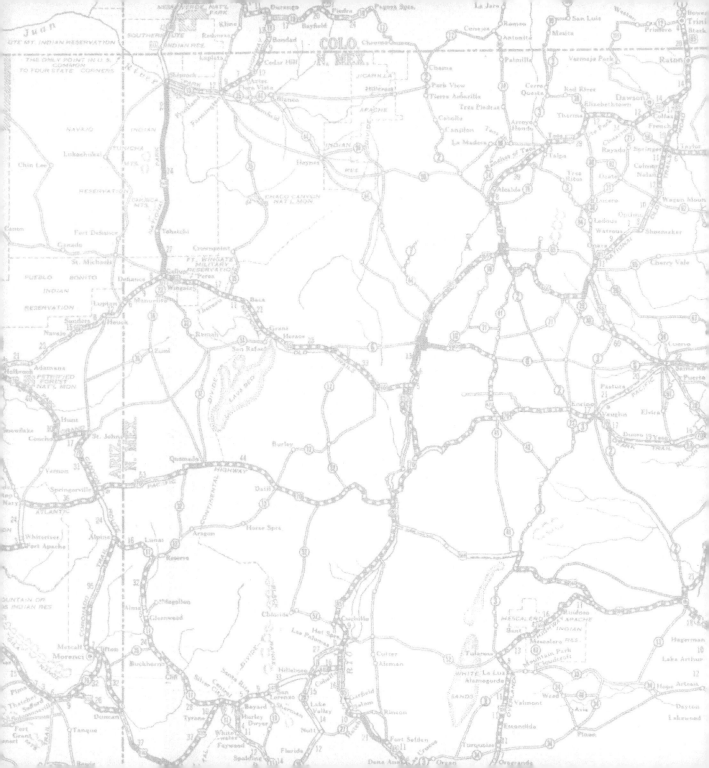

Once More to the Barn

One summer several years ago—during an intermission between moving my mother to a memory care community and an oncoming epoch of personal loss—the bioethicist and author Ruth Levy Guyer invited me to her rented cabin in Maine.

A true friend and a good writer, Ruth had drafted a new book, *A Life Interrupted: The Long Night of Marjorie Day*, the astonishing true story of a woman who lapsed briefly into a coma, remained in an altered state for seventeen years and then suddenly, at midlife, returned to full consciousness, as if she'd just picked up where she'd left off. Though Ruth had meticulously researched her subject ("Daysey," a friend of one of Ruth's friends), she was still working out where and how to insert herself in the narrative, as a medical researcher unraveling this mysterious case. That question is central to the creative nonfiction courses I've taught and to the essays I write, so I was eager to help.

I'd read Ruth's manuscript in one sitting before flying to Bangor, where she and her jovial geneticist husband Mark met me at the airport and drove me to Toddy Pond. Turning pages, marking text, I'd tried not to think of Daysey's story as an allegory of a midlife crisis —this was tough, because her tale is truly stranger than fiction and my mind is a sticky web —but on the road to the cabin, lulled by pleasant conversation and country scenery that made it feel like we were traveling back in time, I thought about my own time away. After seventeen years of raising kids, juggling several jobs and many family crises, I had recently resumed my idled writing career. The publishing industry had drastically changed in the intervening years, and I had changed, too. I was a better writer, but more critical of my work, so I was having trouble adapting to the quick pace and compulsory self-promotion that is the norm today. I couldn't seem to reanimate my younger, more certain self, that literary ingénue for whom death was merely a useful metaphor and not a recurring theme.

Actually, that self had already begun to recede by the time my older daughter was born. In Alison's first baby video, shot by one of Ruth's daughters in the Guyer home, I have shorter hair, greater heft, and new caution as I show off my hearty newborn like evidence against a prenatal hypothesis of fetal neuroblastoma. Ruth was one of the few people I'd told about Alison's abdominal mass, characteristic of this common, often fatal, childhood cancer. Six weeks after her video premiere, a CAT scan would finally confirm my daughter's health. And my brief maternity trauma would retreat to subtext, where every beginning—seasons, friendships, stages of life—resonates with its end.

In the cabin on Toddy Pond, I slept in a twin bed in a room infused with the wet wood scent of decay that, though mundane by now, had alarmed me when I moved east for college from bone-dry Arizona. In the morning, Ruth and I put on sweaters and drank coffee on the dock as we talked about her book, our work, our children, and our parents —deceased (hers) and in decline (mine). The soft morning light turned intense, breakfast blended into lunch, and still we hadn't moved from our chairs. Mark brought us delicious lobster rolls, and then returned to his armchair and his stack of novels.

I love the Guyers. Their daughters, Anya and Dana, are adults now, working in public health and pediatric medicine, but they were my daughters' ages when I met them, enrolled in a summer residential writing program for high school students that I directed at Bryn Mawr College. This fact, though fondly recalled, intruded on the illusion that I was the only child of these excellent parents: science-minded humanists who ask questions and seek answers, who study minute and enormous things, who make meaning from experience. Who live, in other words, as if the world is infinitely worth saving. I felt safe with the Guyers.

Just behind this feeling of safety was a familiar melancholy, a reminder of one generation disappearing into the next—sounding, then fading, throughout the weekend. Within three years, my father and both of my in-laws would die, just as my daughters were leaving home for college. My overwhelming grief at these losses would seem straightforward compared to mourning a loved one living with Alzheimer's disease, a mother who often didn't recognize me.

But talking to my old friend was the best remedy. Ruth had known me before I had children, and so while spending time with her, I could believe that no time had passed at all —that I had just stepped away from myself momentarily and then returned to pick up the thread. Only once was the calm of our long conversation disrupted, when a friendly game warden motor-boated to our dock to boast of the moose he'd tranquilized and transported back to the woods, after it ran amok in a Target parking lot in nearby Ellsworth. He powered up his state-issued laptop and showed us pictures of the poor downed bull. But even that incident was picturesque, a small-town anecdote to bring home to my family.

In Maine, time slowed. It seemed to me that there was still all the time in the world to finish the work I'd barely started—to write down the words that had been trapped in my head while I tended to other life-and-death matters.

That night after dinner, we scraped spoonfuls of ice cream from giant bowls as the field crickets sang outside and moonlight splintered on the tranquil pond. Ruth said, "You know, E.B. White lived near here. He set the county fair in *Charlotte's Web* at the Blue Hill Fairgrounds."

Her words startled me. The children's book is on a personal syllabus I put together gradually over the years as I read to learn how to write—my top-ten list of works that shaped me as a writer and thinker. I knew a bit of White's biography from the flap copy on his children's books and from his widely anthologized essay, "Once More to the Lake." His tribute to *The New Yorker* editor Katharine Sergeant Angell White, "Call Me Ishmael: Or, How I Feel About Being Married to a Bryn Mawr Graduate," is practically required reading at my alma mater. I'd even read his letter to his editor, *Harper & Row's* Ursula Nordstrom, explaining how he came to write about a pig's salvation and why he chose a spider as his hero.

But for all my familiarity with *Charlotte's Web*, I had transposed its Maine setting to the Midwest; in my imagination, White's fictional farm was located in Indiana, where my mother and father were raised. An old black-and-white photo of Mom as a child mingled in my mind with Garth Williams' pen-and-ink drawings of Fern Arable, who saves the runt pig Wilbur from her farmer father's axe. And though I'd never been inside my grandparents' red barn, White had filled in my mental sketch with sensory details from Homer Zuckerman's, where the rescued Wilbur goes to live among sheep, geese, horses, cows, the selfish rat Templeton, and the selfless spider Charlotte.

"That book is one of my favorites," I said to Ruth. "I'd love to see where E.B. White lived while he wrote it." Here was the chance to replant *Charlotte's Web* in its natural soil, I thought, though I kept this to myself. Whatever Ruth's reasons—among them, she's an accommodating host—she quickly agreed to take me there. We planned to visit his home and gravesite before I departed, to pay tribute to the author of the first book that made me cry, and the book that made me believe the right word could save a life.

* * *

The barn was very large. It was very old. It smelled of hay and it smelled of manure. It smelled of the perspiration of tired horses and the wonderful sweet breath of patient cows. It often had a sort of peaceful smell—as though nothing bad could happen ever again in the world.

I first visited Zuckerman's barn in *Charlotte's Web* when I was eight, in the summer of 1971. Trapped inside in triple-digit Phoenix heat, I would have been sprawled across my floral-print bedspread—the fabric antidote to our apartment's Space Age décor—probably chugging a Coke from a slender, pale green bottle and eating a toaster sandwich served on an Atomic Starburst-patterned plate. My parents were at work—they were always at work —selling houses (Mom) and earthmoving machines (Dad) that made the desert habitable for millions of other transplants from the Midwest and the region we Phoenicians called Backeast. My big brother, The Genius, was in his room animating cartoons on a stack of flip pads, while my little brother staged battles with plastic Army men in a theater of war that spanned the moss green carpet in our family room. Our new color television set blared the weekday lineup of game shows, talk shows, reruns of *Star Trek* and *Gilligan's Island,* counting down to the hour when I'd have to put my book away and set the table and start the Hamburger Helper and nag my brother to clear his troops before my parents got home and changed the channel to Walter Cronkite for more dismal news from Vietnam.

Maybe I looked up from White's description of that big old barn reeking of peace to regard our cramped, cluttered apartment in a booming city: air bubbles trapped on the hastily painted walls, icy numbing air conditioning, the windows draped against the sun that incinerated our bland, buff-colored brick apartment building named, without irony, "The Riviera." Compare/contrast. Fantasy/reality. Death as a part of life/life as a living death. Though I wouldn't have put it quite that way back then, I knew which landscape I preferred.

It smelled of grain and of harness dressing and of axle grease and of rubber boots and of new rope. And whenever the cat was given a fish-head to eat, the barn would smell of fish. But mostly it smelled of hay, for there was always hay in the great loft up overhead. And there was always hay being pitched down to the cows and the horses and the sheep.

Besides, White's fictional farm seemed familiar to me, a cultural inheritance from my Hoosier parents, more like home than my actual home. In fact, my business suit-wearing mother still had some Indiana farm girl in her, though she'd left that rustic life behind and embraced mid-century modern architecture and design, instant mashed potatoes, and redundant devices mass-marketed by Ronco.

There were still a few artifacts of her upbringing around: the block of lard (for pie crust) always in our fridge, the sewing patterns abandoned in the back of her closet, her prohibition on cooking chicken or turkey ("filthy animals" she'd seen hopping, headless, around the barnyard), her ban on cats as pets ("too stupid to get out of the way of the combine blades"), and her Republican Party affiliation. Eventually, it emerged that Mom had learned to drive on a tractor. That she knew the difference between hay and straw. That she could detassel corn, cook rhubarb so it tasted good, and roll a tight cigar from whole tobacco leaves. And that, despite her second-wave-feminist career zeal, she felt nostalgic for that farm and for her homegrown, homemade 4-H past.

Nostalgic not in the sense of rosy retrospection, but in the original *nostos algos* sense: pain in going home. Some secret sorrow kept her away; nearly thirty years would pass between the trip I took with her to her oldest brother's funeral and the one my father took with her when she first began losing her memory. On that last journey to Indiana, her childhood home still stood, though the barn had been torn down.

Like any kid, I was curious about my mother's childhood, and wove together details as best I could: odd phrases from my parents' late-night talks; half-conversations from her end of long-distance phone calls; letters tucked into her dresser drawers; slide shows of old photos projected onto a blank wall; my grandmother's visits, which seemed to set the rhythms of Mom's mercurial moods; the *Farmer's Guide Cook Book* my mother inherited when Grandma died.

My grandmother had been a "schoolmarm" before she married my grandfather, who'd served in France in WWI and probably suffered from post-traumatic stress disorder. But it was her post-partum depression that brought the couple and their young sons to Frankfort to be close to her mother. There my grandfather, who'd left a retail management job, reluctantly farmed land adjacent to his in-laws'. Grandma did the best she could— but given her reported misery as a farmwife, finding her recipe for Never Fail Cake Icing, scrawled on a lapsed subscription notice for *The Pathfinder* magazine, brings to mind the scene from *Charlotte's Web*, in which the hired man Lurvy treats Wilbur's existential crisis over his slaughterhouse fate with two spoonfuls of sulphur and a little molasses.

One day not long after Grandma died, Mom brought home a half-peck of heirloom tomatoes, a gift from one of her clients. I'd never tasted a tomato that hadn't come from a can or a cellophane-wrapped tray, so I didn't understand what the big deal was. Nor could I have known the source of her fury when the forgotten fruit ripened and split inside the bag, bleeding juice all over the kitchenette counter and tile floor. But the look on her face was all-too familiar: anger masking grief, screened by her Jackie-O sunglasses.

By the time I actually visited my mother's birthplace as a teenager, the farm in Indiana was no longer just hers, but mine, too; a corresponding landscape had cropped up in my imagination, tilled and seeded and fertilized by many re-readings of *Charlotte's Web*. With each return to the classic fable, Zuckerman's barn morphed further into symbol—until I couldn't read the book without thinking of my mother's lost childhood. I couldn't visit the real-life farm in Frankfort, either, without remembering Zuckerman's barn. The last time I was there, sections of siding from the dismantled barn were stacked in the yard, ready for repurposing. I took a short plank with weathered red paint and the ghost of a horseshoe hanger for a sliding door. The time-worn wood sits on my desk like a totem, the piece somehow conjuring the whole.

Charlotte's Web made me cry for the obvious reasons that Wilbur lives and Charlotte dies. But what really wrecked me—as a kid, and even now—is White's eulogy for his beloved spider, offered in the last two lines: *It is not often that someone comes along who is a true friend and a good writer. Charlotte was both.* At eight, when I tried to picture adulthood, I saw myself sitting at a desk in front of a window, writing with a pencil on paper. This was, I think now, an image of self-possession, and not merely a job. I didn't yet know what I would be when I grew up, but Charlotte—erudite, athletic, resourceful, a devoted friend—was my first model. Charlotte, whose "thin, pleasant" voice first sounds from the darkness of Zuckerman's barn as an answer to baby Wilbur's lonely, anguished tears. Charlotte, who spins a different destiny for the otherwise bacon-bound pig, simply and ingeniously by naming him.

Some Pig.
Terrific.
Radiant.
Humble.

* * *

You remember one thing, and that suddenly reminds you of another thing.

"You could write my life story," my mother said. She was lying on the couch in my childhood home in Phoenix, recovering from the mysterious virus that nearly killed her. I was recovering from her near death, frantically cleaning and making food that she wouldn't eat. Everything tasted bitter to her, including the cigarettes she'd chain-smoked for decades and quit "cold-turkey" when she got sick, as if aversion were self-discipline. She was shrunken and weak, and I was scared. When I'd booked my one-way ticket from Philadelphia to help my father care for her, I feared she'd die before I could get there.

But then one morning, I watched as she hobbled out to the driveway in the late summer heat to peel the Clinton-Gore bumper sticker from my older brother's car, parked there for safekeeping while he was out of town. The idea that this political vandalism would be her last word filled me with existential despair.

"*You* can write your life story," I said.

And yet, I'm the one who keeps returning to Indiana—for weddings, reunions, a cousin's ordination, to scatter my father's ashes, to save my mother's life.

* * *

This is the part of the story where my mother begins to lose her memory. As her history swirls around the existential drain, I give her a pen and paper, like a filter for the residue. "Draw me a map," I say, sitting with her at the kitchen table in the house we moved to when I was twelve. It's been ten years since the near-fatal virus, seven since her second mastectomy, nearly a year since her coronary angioplasty: a stent surgically inserted in the weakened artery that carries blood from her heart. "Of anything. Maybe a place you remember from when you were a kid." The stories she tells about her childhood are always happy.

In black ink, she outlines the ground floor of the house where she was raised: porch, living room, master bedroom, kitchen, utility and storage, breezeway to the coal bin, the cellar beneath. Carefully, she labels rooms and what's inside the rooms, sticking words to arrows, pinning objects to places. *Door, stairs, linen, pot belly stove, bath, toy cupboard, pump, sink, window, lace curtains, cook stove, pantry, electric range, table, piano, Philco radio, porch swing where Bill cried when Fido's puppy got hit by a car.*

"Look more closely at your map," I say. "What interests you the most? Whatever it is, draw it in more detail." Mom says she wants to write about her life, but something's always stopping her. I'm using a prompt that usually works with my creative writing students, trying to find the key that opens the door.

Later, I'll read Michael Sims' *The Story of Charlotte's Web: E.B. White's Eccentric Life in Nature and the Birth of an American Classic* and learn that White began *Charlotte's Web* in a similar way, sketching Zuckerman's barn and yard, and making copious notes on spider behavior. He reportedly suffered from anxiety that was calmed by writing and the company of animals. Anxiety, too, seemed to fuel his story, to infuse it with lovely melancholy: the sad song of late-summer crickets, the weary spider's lonely death. As he wrote to his editor, *A farm is a peculiar problem for a man who likes animals because the fate of most livestock is that they are murdered by their benefactors. It used to be clear to me, slopping a pig, that as far as the pig was concerned I could not be counted on, and this, as I say, troubled me. Anyway, the theme of "Charlotte's Web" is that a pig shall be saved, and I have an idea that somewhere deep inside me there was a wish to that effect.*

Mom continues, drawing the toy cupboard from the kitchen in more detail. Six shelves, divided: "adult junk" up high, "our stuff" within reach. Top: the bottle of castor oil her mother made her take on winter mornings with a slice of orange. Bottom: the doll furniture, empty spools, coloring books, and crayons rattling around in a Sir Walter Raleigh can.

She lingers here.

"Does that cupboard speak to you?" I ask.

"It's inanimate," she says. Though she's asked me for help writing her life story, she thinks what I do is ridiculous. Every Christmas during my "career-building years," she gave me a new business suit, which I saved until the day I finally boxed them up to ship to one of my more sensibly and gainfully employed Indiana cousins.

"Just try," I say.

As she leans into her picture, I see my grandmother there in her place, complaining over her glass of wine and plate of cheese and crackers while Mom smokes in the bathroom and prays for strength. *Sundowning*: we didn't know that word back then. Mom's grandfather was "senile," too, and stopped speaking a decade before he died.

"As you draw, questions might occur to you," I say.

"I don't question objects," she says.

"I don't mean in real life," I say. "I mean in your imagination. Dogs don't really talk, but you like it when I make Froney talk, don't you?" As a kid, I was the ventriloquist for a series of family pets. One of the aspects of *Charlotte's Web* that I've always admired is White's seamless transition from realism to fantasy, first reporting Wilbur's thoughts and then, without fanfare, letting him speak. By the next line, when the goose responds, we've entered a new reality. "Why don't you ask a question?" I urge. "See if the object answers?"

"It doesn't know beans," she says. Then: "Except the rifle. I would not have a gun in my home."

She points to another spot on the map, the porch outside the kitchen door. "That's the fighting place," she says, and I hear familiar, distant rumbling, the violence I've always sensed just outside the picture frame. "My father got out the rifle and threatened to shoot Mother. I remember when I stopped crying *don't!* and said, *Get it over with!*"

"That must have been terrifying," I say.

"I know she drove him to it!" she says. "He loved her more than anything."

I don't know what to do with this. Sometimes memories aren't doors but walls, revealing nothing until the foundation is shaken and the whole house comes down.

"I can't imagine how you survived that," I try.

"I'm strong," she says, and now I know she'll never write this story. As with others she's handed down, she wants me to do it for her—to save her life by preserving it on the page.

A few months before, in summer, I'd driven Mom and my young daughters from Phoenix to Disneyland. On the way, she checked and rechecked her purse for her wallet, her lipstick, the crackers she'd packed. For five hours across that repetitive desert landscape cut through by I-10, she cycled around the same concerns—Where is my wallet? My lipstick? My crackers?—until I started to feel confused, like I'd misheard the question or forgotten the answer. In the backseat, my girls nervously observed this exchange. "Are we there yet?" they asked, over and over again. Then halfway to Anaheim, a storm blew in and we were trapped on the shoulder with a broken windshield wiper as semi-trucks stormed past us at eighty miles an hour. I think I stopped being her daughter then, when Mom looked to me to keep us safe. Finally, the rain stopped. Though I should have turned back, I drove on with the broken wiper, heading into more bad weather you could see coming for miles.

Mom returns to her map, squinting as she fills it in. She traces some parts but not others, as I've instructed her: light for pleasant memories, dark for sad. I've only seen fractions of this farmhouse kitchen in old photos that show long-dead relatives standing at the sink or posing by the back door. But now I imagine that cupboard shimmering in the corner: dark/light, adult/child, chiaroscuro. I see my mother as a little girl, humming to herself while she colors with crayons still smelling of her father's pipe tobacco, making a picture of her happy childhood, the fourth of five children growing up spoiled.

* * *

E.B. White was famously private while he was alive, requesting that journalists only locate him "somewhere on the Atlantic coast," but his 1985 obituary in *The New York Times* finally spilled the beans. The route to his farmhouse in North Brooklin, Maine, is by now well documented, by writers whose real subject seems to be tracking the man to get inside his head. The whole enterprise feels wrong to me, like taking a selfie in a sacred space.

I'll admit that my previous literary pilgrimages with my daughters—what my husband likes to call "The Flinty New England Writers Tour"—weren't planned to inspire reverence for the authors whose homes we visited, but instead, to make them human. I cherished the idea that Alison and Catherine might more freely correspond with Louisa May Alcott, Nathaniel Hawthorne, Ralph Waldo Emerson, Henry David Thoreau, Mark Twain, and Edith Wharton than I could growing up in Arizona, in part because the landscape in which these people lived and wrote would be familiar to them.

When we make a literary pilgrimage, we seek to recover something that's lost: time itself, or wisdom we had once but have misplaced. We seek the dual existence White wrote about in "Once More to the Lake," the overlay of the present on past experience, the child self inside the adult. And, if we're honest, we also look for a souvenir to take home from the site: the barn plank as totem object, a revelatory metaphor, the essay I was already composing in my head as I set out for E.B. White's house with my friend and mentor that morning. Visiting White's home and grave, I was looking for revelation, but I found instead that my lifelong journey through his work had already done the job. Re-reading *Charlotte's Web*, revisiting it with my daughters and my students, I had traveled repeatedly to the place where miracles are performed.

* * *

So, by the time Ruth and I got to Brooklin, the map had been keyed for us and the pilgrim's path cleared: the Blue Hill Inn where White sometimes dined alone after his wife died; the Brooklin Boat Yard where his son Joel (the kid from "Once More to the Lake") and, later, Joel's son Steve worked; the Brooklin General Store, where a teenage cashier gave up the location of his colonial-style farmhouse; down the road, the Brooklin Cemetery where E.B. White is buried beside his beloved Katharine.

Elwyn Brooks White 1899–1985

What's a life, anyway? I thought as I stood by the double headstones, recalling Charlotte's words. *We're born, we live a little, we die.* White was fifty-four when he published his *magnum opus*, seventy-nine when he won the Pulitzer Prize for "his letters, essays, and the full body of his work," eighty-six when he died of Alzheimer's—a disease that, through destruction, reveals the mundane miracle of the intact mind, which functions like a graceful spider practicing her trapping and philological skills.

Charlotte offered her friend Wilbur a glimmer of hope as she patiently waited for a plan to come to her. I know that feeling viscerally now: the beating wings of an idea on the verge of being caught. And after a long period of quietly thinking, Charlotte's elegant solution to Wilbur's plight—the words she'd weave into her web to elevate the poor, doomed pig —finally arrived as the summer was half gone and the crickets began sounding their alarm, alerting her to her deadline.

* * *

I've pilgrimaged through *Charlotte's Web* dozens of times by now, more than any other book on my shelves. When I pick up my original copy, its pages brittle and browning, it falls open to the chapter titled "Escape." And I return once more to the barn, where *there was always hay in the great loft up overhead. And there was always hay being pitched down to the cows and the horses and the sheep.* I think about the beauty of that single image, one of so many in the book: the harvested grass hoisted aloft in the barn and then pitched down to earth again as sustenance. In art class at her memory care community, my mother paints the red barn over and over again. At my desk in front of the window, I begin to write by asking: What keeps us alive and what will our deaths feed?

Always Home
for Christmas

Hark! the herald angels sang throughout my childhood in Phoenix, whenever *The Glorious Sound of Christmas* played on my parents' hi-fi. Fourteen songs performed by The Philadelphia Orchestra and the Temple University Concert Choir. Forty-five minutes of satin sound, from a treasure box that opened with trumpet fanfare and closed with the hushed choir singing a solemn "Silent Night, Holy Night."

This album of familiar carols and rarely recorded sacred songs was my favorite, if an unlikely soundtrack to our 1970s southwestern celebrations. For us, Christmas was sunshine and sombreroed Santas, saguaro cacti wrapped in white lights and paper bag luminarias lining our street, enchiladas on Christmas eve—and this glorious music with its polished, seamless Philadelphia sound. I'd lie on the shag carpet near our fake fir (real trees are fire hazards in the dry climate) listening to Beethoven's "The Worship of God" or Schubert's "Ave Maria," and forget to tally my presents or fight my brothers for the last Mexican wedding cake. I loved the whole record, but these pieces in particular transported me to a different, distant landscape I'd never actually seen: sparkling snow, stone spire against a dark sky, warm candlelight reflected in stained-glass windows. My family didn't go to church. To me, that music—grand and powerful, filling the room, making me feel full—was church.

Going gold at its debut in 1962, *The Glorious Sound of Christmas* sold more than a million copies that season; it was "one of the fastest-selling classical sets in history" according to the Record Industry Association of America. By then, conductor Eugene

Ormandy and his orchestra were already famous far beyond Philly, thanks to radio broadcasts, numerous recordings, and a concert on CBS—the first-ever televised symphonic orchestra performance. This may explain how their new Christmas album made its way into so many households like mine, where the classical music we recognized came mostly from Disney's *Fantasia*, Warner Brothers cartoons, and my mother's piano. The year I was born, that widely beloved record joined a cacophonous canon of holiday music of the era, including *Christmas with the Chipmunks*, Bing Crosby's *I Wish You a Merry Christmas*, and Vince Guaraldi's *A Charlie Brown Christmas*. And there it stayed, played on various devices (for LP, cassette, mp3, compact disc) for more than fifty years as the album was reborn and remixed, getting scratched and warped and, eventually, replaced when technology advanced or the recording wore out.

* * *

But traditions, like canons, change.

The first time I took my young daughters to The Philadelphia Orchestra's annual holiday concert at the new Kimmel Center, they couldn't understand why I was so moved. They were too young to sense the overlay of present on past experience, or to know how the child self folds into the adult. They were listening to pretty music, while I marveled that the Christmas that music conjured when I was a kid is now the version I live.

This year, my husband and I choose concert tickets in the third tier, third row, center. As empty nesters, we don't need to see the stage, though it's beautifully decorated with trees and wreaths and red and green lights. We sit where, in that cello-shaped hall, the music sounds best. Over the years, we've heard The Philadelphia Orchestra and The Mendelssohn Club of Philadelphia under several conductors. Tonight's Bramwell Tovey is less guest than host, inviting the audience into a light, festive program that harks back to the old album with just two of its songs: "Hark! The Herald Angels Sing" and "O Come, All Ye Faithful."

People love it. Around us, the audience—in jeans and party dresses, athletic shoes and polished loafers with argyle socks—laugh at Tovey's music jokes and, with his encouragement, clap along to "Sleigh Ride." He pays tribute to Ormandy and his orchestra's gold standard of Christmas albums, but this is really Tovey's show: a program of his jazzy arrangements and a

"Rittenhouse Carol" he composed. And he's truly wonderful—especially as he recites "A Visit from St. Nicholas" while playing piano for a medley bookended by "Santa Claus is Coming to Town."

"This is the most fun orchestra in America!" he exclaims, promoting the musicians as Ormandy did on the radio during my parents' childhoods. "And they're here every week!"

People come to a holiday concert with a different set of ears, Tovey has said, and the trick to pleasing an audience is playing the music people know. That's why I'm overcome every time I put on *The Glorious Sound of Christmas* and that first trumpet sounds. I have memorized Arthur Harris's arrangements—every bell, every trumpet, every soaring violin. That album, for me, is an artifact of a particular place and time that I can't return to, except through music.

To be embraced by my husband's family was to be absorbed into their traditions and gradually, unintentionally, to give up most of mine. For years, we travelled between Arizona and Maryland, warm weather and cold, the rowdy excess of my family and the polite restraint of his. Now it seems we've settled here, setting the table with his grandmother's china, serving hard sauce for plum pudding in my mother-in-law's red enamel dish, attending a candlelight church service and singing carols. It's quite like the picture I imagined once, but all I can think of is home.

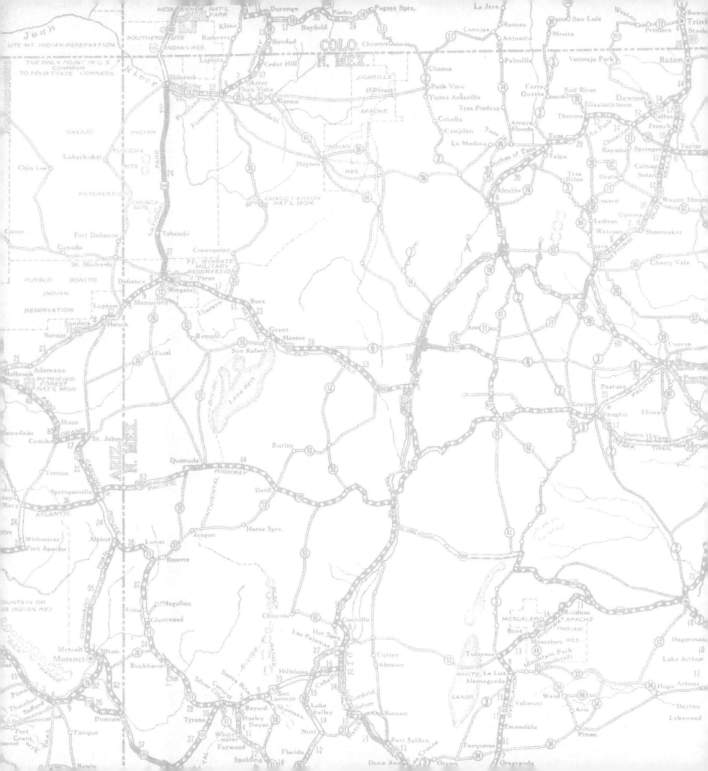

Believers

The sauceboat showed up in a bag of filthy artifacts dug up at Philadelphia's National Constitution Center site. To my untrained eye, it was just another dirty dish for a volunteer technician like me to wash, label, and catalogue. But judging from the buzz in the archaeology lab the day the ceramics collector visited, this piece was important, even precious.

Independence National Historical Park archaeologists believed they'd unearthed a colonial-era treasure: an intact example of Bonnin and Morris soft-paste porcelain made by the American China Manufactory in the Southwark section of the city. Corroded and discolored, the sauceboat didn't resemble the company's nineteen known surviving pieces (sauceboats, tiny baskets, pickle dishes, and stands) exhibited at the Philadelphia Museum of Art. Tests to determine its chemical structure were inconclusive and the underglaze blue-painted decoration was gone, but the sauceboat was the right shape and bore the right factory mark. If authentic, it was historically significant: a souvenir from the campaign to sell locally-produced ceramics to colonists, which lasted until Josiah Wedgwood flooded the market with cheap imported English porcelain in the testy years leading up to the Revolutionary War.

But history was only half of it; something else seemed to be at stake. As I inked field specimen numbers onto a seemingly endless pile of pottery sherds, the collector toured the lab. He boasted about valuable acquisitions and revealed his inexperience with mending artifacts to a team of archaeologists who routinely put together shattered vessels like a novelist fits words. His tone and swagger reminded me of an English professor who'd once told me casually—not expecting an argument—that creative work is validated by criticism. As if making meaning wasn't the purpose of writing fiction; as if the point of archaeology was to display objects in a glass case, and not to learn about the people who used them.

With an exasperated sigh, the collector dismissed treasure seekers who hoped against his expert appraisals that what they'd found in Grandma's attic was worth something.

"Believers!" he said.

Bingo, I thought.

With a word, he'd unmasked himself. Though the archaeologists might never know if the sauceboat was a true Bonnin and Morris, uncertainty wouldn't change their work. And yet the collector had discounted these cultural stewards, who sift through our soil and process every last seed and bone and bead, and who must temper the critic's urge to curate with the creator's habit of curiosity. Believers, indeed: archaeologists and artists will spend our lives searching because the process of searching is valuable.

Like any object, the sauceboat means something different to every person who encounters it. For the collector, the thing itself is valuable, both for its scarcity and its arcanum, the trade-secret recipe for turning coarse elements such as glass and bone and soapstone into fine porcelain. For the archaeologists, the object's importance is partly its provenience, which provides an important context clue. British-born Gousse Bonnin and Philadelphian George Anthony Morris were in business for only two years; the manufacturers' narrow production window (1770–72) helps date other artifacts found in the same strata, on a time-line moving backwards from the contemporary surface to the deep past.

For me, the object conjures Thanksgiving—not my elegant adult remake of the holiday, but the dismal childhood version I remember: my family awkward in dress-up clothing, arguing and blasting aerosol cheese onto Ritz crackers while a turkey roasts interminably, filling the house with the sad smell of sage. My family of origin is my personal arcanum, an alchemy of resentment and grief that rendered me smooth and brittle. Memories are my material. Writing is the way I keep myself from shattering.

My point is that we value objects (or not) according to the personal meaning that we bestow. Perhaps it's sacrilegious to say it, but since the sauceboat's discovery, I've often wondered if the pristine Bonnin and Morris pickle stand I viewed in its case in Gallery 286 of the Philadelphia Museum of Art escaped the privy pit not because it was treasured, but because it is absurd. In life as in memory, what we don't use is preserved intact—while the archaeological record is often created in crisis, with emotion guiding what we take with us and what we leave behind.

I speak from some experience. In the seven years I've spent volunteering at the archaeology lab, I've emptied four houses full of objects collected by declining parents and departed parents-in-law. Though Thanksgiving dinner china was abundantly represented, it never once made any sibling's must-have list. I gave away fancy serving pieces to the Goodwill in my hometown, and donated dishes, flatware, and pots and pans to the Nationalities Service Center in Philadelphia, to help furnish the homes of refugees recently arrived here from all over the world. For myself, I claimed items with personal value: my mother's measuring spoons, my grandmother's cook book, the wooden doll cradle my father made for me, my old softball glove, my mother-in-law's trove of craft supplies. These small, forgotten things are like the fingerprints potters leave in the clay: evidence of the maker in what lost family members finished or hoped to finish one day.

When my beloved mother-in-law died, the apartment seemed even quieter with the noise of unstrung beads clicking together in drawers, and fat spools of colorful quilting thread rolling from side to side in wooden trays. There were boxes and boxes of fabric still scented with her drugstore perfume and permeated with the sadness of things left undone. Overwhelmed, I emailed my friend Marta Maretich in London, who quilts as brilliantly as she writes. I knew that Marta—whose own fabric stash she describes as "the size of a large, well-fed sow, packed in a plaid plastic bag with handles, the kind you see on the news in Asian refugee situations"—would know what to do.

"What would I keep?" she responded, in a message I read in the wee hours with relief and gratitude. "This is the practical me talking: all pure cottons, all solids, even dull, muddy ones because they make a useful contrast with brights. Anything geometric, anything really vintage. Anything seasonal, because even when you don't think you'll ever use a poinsettia print, you find yourself needing one. Orange fabrics are oddly useful in many situations, not least at Halloween. Scraps from things she made for you, because you will use them in your own projects and think of her. Fabrics that remind you of her for any reason whatsoever. Green fabrics, because you love green—there should be plenty in the stash, because undoubtedly she knew you loved green, too."

It was exactly what I needed to hear to get through the heartbreak of breaking ground. As I worked my way through the fabric, I mourned my mother-in-law, but I felt hopeful, too. The heirloom quilt I plan to piece together from her remnants will be a rare accomplishment, given my meager sewing skills. It won't be anything a collector would want, but it will comfort my daughters in incalculable ways long after I am gone.

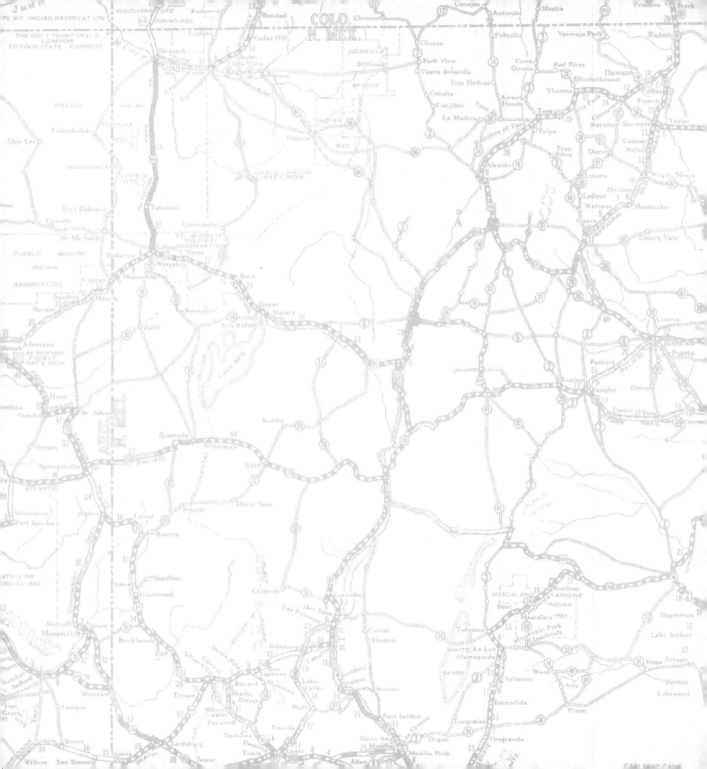

Acknowledgements

I gratefully acknowledge these publications, in which versions of these essays originally appeared:

Cleaver: "Believers"

Creative Nonfiction: "The Pit and the Page"

Hunger Mountain: "Primary Sources"

1966: A Journal of Creative Nonfiction: "I Have, I Fear, the Literary Temperament" and "Memorial"

The Philadelphia Inquirer: "Art and Artifact," "The Social Life of Maps," and "Always Home for Christmas"

You Are Here: the Journal of Creative Geography: "The Big Tree, Phoenix, Arizona"

I would like to thank Independence National Historical Park archaeologists Jed Levin, Deborah Miller, and Willie Hoffman for their painstaking stewardship of our nation's artifacts and the stories these treasures tell. As a volunteer technician in the archaeology lab, I benefitted directly from their passion for urban archaeology and their patience with my many questions. Thanks, too, to the talented Thursday volunteer crew—Dick and Nancy Grove, Randy Rosensteel, and Carolyn Scott—for seven years of conversation and camaraderie.

Huge thanks to Elliott Shore for inviting me into his course on the history of Bryn Mawr College, and to Eric Pumroy and the Special Collections staff at Bryn Mawr for their expert guidance in the archives.

I am fortunate to work with enthusiastic editors, who coaxed this book into existence with assignments and acceptances, especially *Cleaver* founding editor Karen Rile, and Avery Rome and Kevin Ferris at *The Philadelphia Inquirer*, who gave me column space to share my interests in Philadelphia culture and history. Finally, my heartfelt gratitude to Nayt Rundquist and the New Rivers Press staff and student interns for bringing this book home.

About the Author

Elizabeth Mosier logged one thousand volunteer hours processing colonial-era artifacts at Philadelphia's Independence National Historical Park Archeology Laboratory to write *Excavating Memory: Archaeology and Home*. A graduate of Bryn Mawr College and the MFA Program for Writers at Warren Wilson College, her nonfiction work has been selected as notable in *Best American Essays* and appears widely in journals and newspapers including *Cleaver*, *Creative Nonfiction*, and *The Philadelphia Inquirer*. She writes the "Intersections" column for the *Bryn Mawr Alumnae Bulletin*.

About New Rivers Press

New Rivers Press emerged from a drafty Massachusetts barn in winter 1968. Intent on publishing work by new and emerging poets, founder C.W. "Bill" Truesdale labored for weeks over an old Chandler & Price letterpress to publish three hundred fifty copies of Margaret Randall's collection *So Many Rooms Has a House but One Roof*. About four hundred titles later, New Rivers is now a nonprofit learning press, based since 2001 at Minnesota State University Moorhead. Charles Baxter, one of the first authors with New Rivers, calls the press "the hidden backbone of the American literary tradition."

As a learning press, New Rivers guides student editors, designers, writers, and filmmakers through the various processes involved in selecting, editing, designing, publishing, and distributing literary books. In working, learning, and interning with New Rivers Press, students gain integral real-world knowledge that they bring with them into the publishing workforce at positions with publishers across the country, or to begin their own small presses and literary magazines.

Please visit our website: newriverspress.com for more information.